PENGU

natural men's health

PENELOPE SACH is Australia's leading practitioner of naturo-pathic, homoeopathic and herbal medicine. She runs a highly successful clinic in Sydney and produces her own range of organically grown herbal teas. Her most recent book was *Natural Woman*.

For more about Penelope Sach,
visit www.penelopesach.com.au

Other titles by Penelope Sach

Healing and Cleansing with Herbal Tea
Natural Woman
Detox
The Little Book of Wellbeing
Take Care of Yourself

natural
men's health

PENELOPE
SACH

PENGUIN BOOKS

Penguin Books

Published by the Penguin Group
Penguin Books Australia Ltd
250 Camberwell Road, Camberwell, Victoria 3124, Australia
Penguin Books Ltd
80 Strand, London WC2R 0RL, England
Penguin Putnam Inc.
375 Hudson Street, New York, New York 10014, USA
Penguin Books, a division of Pearson Canada
10 Alcorn Avenue, Toronto, Ontario, Canada M4V 3B2
Penguin Books (NZ) Ltd
Cnr Rosedale and Airborne Roads, Albany, Auckland, New Zealand
Penguin Books (South Africa) (Pty) Ltd
24 Sturdee Avenue, Rosebank, Johannesburg 2196, South Africa
Penguin Books India (P) Ltd
11, Community Centre, Panchsheel Park, New Delhi 110 017, India

First published by Penguin Books Australia Ltd 2003

1 3 5 7 9 10 8 6 4 2

Cover design by Susannah Low and Judith Grace, Penguin Design Studio
Text design by Susannah Low, Penguin Design Studio
Cover photograph © Julie Anne Renouf
Typeset in ITC Legacy Serif by Post Pre-press Group, Brisbane, Queensland
Printed and bound in Australia by McPherson's Printing Group, Maryborough, Victoria

National Library of Australia
Cataloguing-in-Publication data:

Sach, Penelope.
Natural men's health.

Includes index.
ISBN 0 14 100385 5.

1. Men – Health and hygiene. 2. Men – Physiology. 3. Men – Diseases. I. Title.

613.0423

www.penguin.com.au

To my father
Alan Ivens Sach

✳ Contents

Introduction

This book has been written because of the increasing number of men who come through my door seeking advice for complaints which are either specific to or have particular effects on men.

There are many differences between men and women, and one of the areas in which this is most obvious is in the way they deal with health issues. Most men are impatient with illness, especially their own. They don't have time to be slowed down by bad health and want to resolve problems quickly.

What I have also observed about men, both as clients and as friends, is that it often takes a little time for them to change unhealthy lifestyle habits. I think part of the reason for this is that it takes them a while to admit to having a problem. On the other hand, once they accept that there is a health issue that needs to be dealt with and decide to make a change, they can become quite obsessive. On the whole, men are very driven by goals and once they're on a roll, there is no stopping them.

In my private practice, I have treated many men but I have noticed a particular upsurge of interest in men's health over the last five years. Certainly, when I first began my practice in the mid-80s, the vast majority of my clients were women and children. It wasn't until the 90s that the husbands of the women I treated started being sent to me – some willingly and some reluctantly! These men were not 'new age' men. They were from all walks of life: businessmen, tradesmen, athletes, lawyers – even a few doctors! Many of these men had already been down the orthodox medicine path and come away very disillusioned. So often they had been told 'You must lose weight' or 'You need to cut down your stress', but they were never given any advice on how to do this.

The more men I treated, the more I began to investigate and understand the particular health needs of men. I was thrilled to be able to use the principles of diet, nutrition, plant medicine and vitamins to assist them with the ever-increasing number of problems they discussed with me.

Natural medicine was never meant to take the place of orthodox medicine. It offers an alternative approach and provides ideas for preventing health problems. Supporting the systems of your body in times of lowered immunity, stress or poor digestion is a far better option than reaching for a quick-fix remedy of antibiotics or a headache pill.

Many men have cottoned on to the fact that diet and lifestyle management, as well as naturopathic treatments and supplements, will give them the good health and, above all, the energy to flourish in the face of stress, long work hours and all the modern complications of relationships and life in the 21st century.

The world is changing and so are we. Life expectancy is greater and everyone's lives seem to be getting busier. But greater awareness of how our bodies tick and what we put into them can help us deal with the stresses of life. Possibly this book can help you recognise potential for change in your life.

No one has a great deal of time to read lengthy books about the chemistry of health. In this book, I have set out to give you an understanding of what has worked consistently in treating common men's health complaints – but it's only the tip of the iceberg. Enjoy the book and use it as a reference. Try the ideas and make small changes over a period of time. You'll be amazed at how much better you will feel.

NOTE: For each condition or symptom I have recommended a series of supplements. The most effective way of using this book is to take just the first one or two supplements listed for the first few weeks. These are the most important herbs and vitamins for dealing with your condition. If you feel better after taking these and want to continue your improvement, then add to your regime from the other recommended supplements.

I have also included suggested dosages for most of the recommended herbs and vitamins. Many of them come in standard dosages at your health store and you should always check the label to see exactly what you're getting. If in doubt, please ask your naturopath or health-store assistant. (See also *How to buy supplements*, page 190.)

1
Digestion

Digestive problems are probably one of the most common health concerns for men today. Despite the fact that many men think they're just something they have to live with, the good news is that common complaints such as acid stomach, heartburn, irregular bowel motions, flatulence and general digestive discomfort can all be radically improved. An acidic environment in the digestive tract is the most common reason for these complaints.

The main causes of acid build-up in the digestive system are:

- poor digestion
- overeating
- an excess of refined carbohydrates, including white flour and refined sugar products
- a lack of fresh fruit and vegetables daily.

I have treated many men with these digestive problems over the years; 90 per cent respond extraordinarily well to simple changes in diet, and some general knowledge of what is actually happening to their digestive system. Food can broadly be divided into two groups: acid and alkaline, and it is vital that the digestive system has 60–70 per cent alkaline foods daily and only 30 per cent acidic foods to prevent common digestive problems. Sticking to this split will also increase vitality.

Acid creators – the negatives for digestion
- Refined sugar and white flour products
- Red meat
- Alcohol and stress also have a negative impact on digestion and can be classed as acid creators.

Alkaline creators – the positives for digestion
- Fresh fruit and vegetables
- All raw juices, especially carrot, watermelon and green vegetable juices (spinach, the top of beetroot leaves and wheat grass)
- Herbal teas
- Unpasteurised honey
- Raw almonds

- Miso soup
- Tofu
- Sea vegetables
- Lima and adzuki beans (other beans, except for those which are soaked and have sprouted, are acidic)
- Fresh deep-sea fish, such as flake, blue grenadier, orange roughy or John Dory (these are the least acid-forming protein you can include in your diet, apart from legumes which should be included with vegetables to balance an acid stomach).

CASE STUDY

A man aged 57 visited me in 1995 for a check-up and general health advice. His energy levels were low and he had stopped smoking one month before seeing me. He felt that his digestion was not right and he had been suffering a bloated stomach. He also complained of fungus around his toes.

I suggested he follow a diet for three months that was yeast-free and also free of acidic foods, such as orange juice, wine and tomatoes, and carbohydrates such as bread, pasta and cheese, which contain a high amount of yeast. I also gave him a tonic to assist liver detoxification and recommended an anti-oxidant tablet with an omega 3 and 6 oil capsule twice a day.

After three weeks, he returned feeling much better. His bloating had eased and he said that the tonic had really made a difference. He continued with the tonic for another four months. I now see him once a year and although he is not completely strict with his diet, he knows what to do when he feels digestive problems come on and returns to me for a top-up of his tonic for two to three months.

If you have severe symptoms relating to your digestive system, such as continual diarrhoea or pain in the stomach or bowel, a doctor can run some tests. For example, testing for the presence of a bacteria called *Helicobacter pylori* requires a simple breath test, which your local doctor can do. If the test is positive, the treatment generally takes the form of a specialised medication for a few days. The patient is then asked to have another breath test to see if the bacteria has been eliminated. The presence of *Helicobacter pylori* bacteria in the gut has been found to cause long-term problems throughout the body if not treated. It can lead to ulcers, irritable bowel syndrome and cancer. I recommend that men have a test to check for helicobacter if they have poor digestion, bad breath or irregular bowel movements.

Bowel polyps are also common in men. If you have a family history of polyps, then it is advisable to have a regular colonoscopy. It is known that polyps in the bowel can lead to bowel cancer. Likewise, if there is a history of bowel cancer or any major cancer to do with the digestive system in your family, then you should discuss precautionary tests with your doctor.

CASE STUDY

I advised a man of 60 to investigate the state of his bowel with a colonoscopy as his iris showed signs of bowel toxicity. (To a naturopath, the iris is a good indicator of the state of certain organs of the body.) He had no symptoms of irregular bowel motions or gas but his taste for alcohol had definitely taken its toll on the bowel wall causing an acid environment and revealing a dark circle around the bowel area of the iris. He rang me a few weeks later to say the specialist had found four polyps, which were removed immediately.

As a preventative to acid build-up I prescribed slippery elm bark capsules, two before breakfast and dinner, and also at lunch if he was drinking alcohol. I also advised taking an anti-oxidant tablet and omega oil capsule daily.

There are now a number of studies suggesting that general bowel problems, often referred to as 'leaky gut' may be linked to poor concentration. In this case, a naturopath can assist in correcting bowel flora and repairing the permeability of the gut wall. A liver detox can also help.

*Heartburn (indigestion)

Heartburn is a burning sensation felt behind the breastbone following eating. The condition is caused by the reflux of gastric contents into the oesophagus and is often referred to as reflux oesophagitis. In many instances, the condition can be improved radically simply by changing the diet and taking some herbal supplements.

It is ridiculous to take antacid medication continually without looking into the problem and trying to solve it. Follow the suggested dietary changes set out on page 13 and see if your condition improves. If it doesn't, I suggest you consult a specialist who can do an endoscopy to have a look at your stomach and oesophageal lining.

CASE STUDY

In my practice, I have treated many men who have complained of problems with indigestion, heartburn and fatigue. Many of them often follow a sensible diet already, including lots of vegetables and salad, so changes in this area are not necessarily the answer. I do suggest that they cut down their intake of fatty foods and also advise that they eat regular meals. I encourage them to eat a variety of rice and protein dishes or simple healthy sandwiches for lunch.

I recently saw a builder who suffers from heartburn. He had skipped breakfast and lunch for many years, often only eating a piece of fruit at these times. He was given medication by his specialist but he came to me to discuss changing his diet.

Because he complained of feeling sick in the mornings (he had a 5 a.m. start each day), I suggested he start the day with just a glass of water. At 9 a.m., I suggested having one or two sandwiches with chicken or tuna and salad. I also gave him a soy protein powder which he mixed into a large glass of water and drank three to four times a day for energy and to soothe the oesophagus.

When he returned to see me four weeks later, he was maintaining his new regime very strictly and felt so much better for it. His heartburn had improved and he had stopped his medication (under the doctor's instructions). I advised him to stay on the program for another three months.

Treatment & prevention program

▓ Cut out all acidic foods such as wine, orange juice, tomato juice, cheese, beer, citrus fruits, white sugar and processed and prepackaged food. Do this for at least six weeks to see an improvement. Then slowly reintroduce a few acidic foods once every second or third day.

▓ Eat regularly and avoid leaving the stomach empty for longer than four hours. In fact, it is ideal to have a snack in between meals, even if it is just a banana.

▓ Try to eat simple foods that are gentle on the stomach. Porridge in the morning is ideal, and mashed potato and soup are great to incorporate into your daily diet. Cooked vegetables are more soothing to the stomach than salads.

Supplements

Sometimes vitamins can upset the digestive system so it's always best to check with your naturopath or health professional before taking any vitamins.

Try slippery elm bark powder or capsules as this herb is soothing and healing to the irritated lining of the digestive system. It is referred to as a mucilagenous herb as it is sticky when mixed with warm water, and if taken before eating it protects against inflammation of the oesophagus. It is safe for long-term use. The powder is better than the capsules in the first month of treatment. When mixing the powder, stir a teaspoonful quickly in warm water and drink within 6–8 seconds, otherwise the mixture will coagulate. The capsules are ideal at lunch if it's inconvenient for you to mix the powder.

Slippery elm bark is also great to use as a preventative in times of stress, when you may produce extra acid in the stomach. It is one of the best herbs available to keep the bowel regular and stop acid building up after eating refined foods. Take two to three capsules before each meal. Take the same dose before bed if you have heartburn. Continue until your condition improves.

✳Irritable bowel and stomach ulcers

Irritable bowel means that there is some damage or irritation to the lining of the bowel wall (referred to as the mucosal lining). This needs to be repaired by eating gentle foods, eliminating food allergies and irritants, and gently incorporating some herbs and vitamins into the diet. This can be done slowly by adding a supplement a week.

Many men are diagnosed with irritable bowel and generally there is little that the medical profession can do except prescribe long-term antacids or small amounts of steroids. The symptoms include irregular bowel movements varying from constipation to diarrhoea. Flatulence, acid reflux and allergies to some foods are also common in those who have this condition.

Dietary changes are vital and a diet heavily weighted with alkaline foods is critical in treating this condition (see suggested diet on pages 16–18).

Stomach ulcers (peptic ulcers) and duodenal ulcers can often occur on a diet high in acidic foods and/or when meals have been consistently irregular. The presence of *Helicobacter pylori* has been found to be the biggest cause of ulcers in the digestive tract.

Ulcers are often painful. It is imperative that a doctor checks them; preferably the patient should be referred to a gastro-enterologist. If ulcers are found, then medication will be prescribed for the short term.

A major part of my work involves the prevention and ongoing treatment of ulcers. The stomach and digestive tract must be kept healthy so that unwanted bacteria cannot breed. A balanced diet is critical.

The body suffers under the strain of poor digestion, ulcers and an inflamed bowel, and taking the supplements suggested on pages 19–20 will boost your energy levels enormously.

Treatment & prevention program

The following is a suggested dietary plan. Dietary changes can be made while on medication.

Breakfast

❊ Porridge with low-fat milk. If you are allergic to dairy milk or have mucus problems, use soy milk or rice milk.

❊ Cereal accompanied by a milkshake with a tablespoon of a good protein powder. The protein assists in rebuilding the damaged cells in the lining of the digestive system and assists an acid stomach.

❊ Toast with two boiled eggs.

Lunch and dinner

❊ A sandwich filled with some form of protein such as chicken, turkey, tuna or salmon. If you have salad with your sandwich, do not include tomatoes until your condition improves. Do not add vinegar to green salad – use only olive oil.

❊ A rice dish with a protein and cooked vegetables, but make sure the dish is not loaded with additives, which can aggravate the condition. For this reason, avoid takeaway Chinese and Thai food.

❄ If you're eating out in a restaurant, minestrone soup is a good option as it will assist an acid stomach. Then, if possible, choose fish or chicken (do not eat too much red meat as it needs acid to break it down) with three cooked vegetables.

Avoid

❄ Nuts, chilli and foods that are heavily laced with additives. They will upset the bowel.

❄ Alcohol for four to six weeks and then only gin and tonic, or brandy or vodka for another four to six weeks.

❄ Vitamin C, which can upset the system after an ulcer.

Generally, a doctor will give you medication for an ulcer but it is essential to adopt, alongside the medication, a simple allergy-free and non-irritant diet as described above.

Supplements

- One vitamin E 500 IU tablet after each meal. This wonderful anti-oxidant specifically helps the healing of the membrane wall in the digestive tract. If you have high blood pressure, check the dosage with your doctor.

- A soy protein powder or a whey protein powder. This is very helpful in the first six weeks of healing an ulcer. You can take this powder three times a day between meals. Add a tablespoon to a large glass of water or skim milk. Blend it like a shake or just put the powder in and stir if you are at work. If you are drinking alcohol (although it's preferable to exclude it altogether), then take this powder beforehand and try to avoid wine and stick to herb-based spirits.

- One to two boswellia tablets twice a day. This herb is brilliant for those with irritable bowel. It prevents the inflammation usually present in this condition and, taken on a regular basis, it can be curative.

- One teaspoon of aloe vera juice twice a day for a few months. This is an excellent substance that helps repair the mucosal lining of the bowel.

- My Triple E tea made from pure liquorice root throughout the day. Liquorice has natural anti-inflammatory properties. (Not to be confused with liquorice lollies which are flavoured sugar with a few drops of aniseed!)

- Slippery elm bark capsules or powder: two capsules or a heaped teaspoon in warm water twice daily. This can help prevent the development of new ulcers and should be taken long term.

- A teaspoon of acidophilus powder in a glass of water before breakfast and dinner to restore the natural bowel flora. By doing this, symptoms of flatulence and bloating are reduced. This is especially important for those who have taken antibiotics long term.

✳ Gallstones

Gallstones form in the gall bladder, which sits just under the liver on the right side of the body. The gall bladder is responsible for processing bile, which is originally made in the liver and then moves through the gall bladder to continue the elimination of toxins and the breakdown of fats.

If this organ becomes overloaded through poor diet and lots of toxins, then it will not digest fats properly. The symptoms of an overloaded gall bladder include nausea, headaches and the vomiting of bile. These symptoms can also indicate that gallstones are present. An ultrasound by your doctor can confirm the diagnosis.

✳ CASE STUDY

A 75-year-old man came to visit me for a check-up. He had always taken vitamins and lived a very active life playing golf three times a week and tennis once a week. When I looked at the vitamins and dosages he was taking, I realised that he was doubling up on several things. It is much better to take a single tablet with a higher and more suitable dose than many tablets with a lower dose. This is generally easier on the system as well as the hip pocket.

It wasn't until a year later that he came to me complaining of nausea and bloating. I suspected gallstones and suggested he ask his doctor to refer him for an ultrasound. Many small stones showed up. He was keen to treat them through dietary changes and his doctor was happy to go along with this.

I gave him a tonic to assist the breakdown of the stones and to help his liver and gallbladder with the secretion of bile. I also discovered (via his wife) that he had a sweet tooth and regularly ate cake or biscuits in the afternoon. I suggested he substitute fruit for this. I also prescribed two slippery elm bark capsules before breakfast and dinner to ease his bloating.

He is now doing very well and has also lost some weight. Now, after eight months, he only takes the tonic once a day or when he feels he needs to.

I've often noticed that many men who have an intolerance to fatty foods and a history of gallstones in the family can have gallstones themselves without suffering many severe symptoms. In this case, I often suggest taking a tablet of St Mary's thistle daily to assist the liver.

If you do not have stones but do have a sluggish gall bladder, your naturopath can help.

Treatment & prevention program

If gallstones are present, your doctor will probably recommend their removal, or the removal of the entire gall bladder, especially if the stones are large and are causing other significant problems such as nausea, migraines and a lack of vitality.

If the stones are smaller in size and you feel unwell, with digestive upsets such as heartburn, mild headaches and discomfort after eating fatty foods, then I recommend the following.

※ Avoid fried foods and milk or other dairy products in your diet.

※ Take omega 3 oils, one capsule three times a day or three capsules once a day. This assists in bile and fat metabolism.

⚒ Have a herbal tonic made from fluid extract or tincture of each of the following: fringe tree (20%), dandelion root (20%), barberry (20%), peppermint (10%), hydrastis (10%) and St Mary's thistle (20%). Take half a teaspoon after each meal and when the digestion is upset or 30–40 drops in quarter of a glass of water three times a day. This tonic helps to slowly break down smaller stones.

⚒ If you are unable to find this tonic, buy a tablet made from some of the plants above, or just use St Mary's thistle over a long term (twelve months): one tablet after each meal.

✳ Kidney stones

Men who suffer from kidney stones tell me that when they pass the stone the pain is excruciating. We don't totally understand why kidney stones form. The problem can be inherited, caused by poor diet, or set off by an imbalance in calcium metabolism.

I have noticed that most men who suffer from kidney stones do not drink enough water. The kidneys are not properly flushed which encourages an environment where the stones develop.

Treatment & prevention program

▓ Drink two litres of water daily.

▓ Have a tonic containing equal parts of the following herbs: cornsilk, crateva, marshmallow, buchu, uva-ursi, echinacea and nettle. Take one teaspoon three times a day or 7 ml twice a day in a glass of water (200 ml).

▓ Eliminate coffee altogether and drink alcohol in moderation, for six weeks.

▓ Drink two glasses of cranberry juice each day. Make sure you obtain a very good quality product from a health store.

✳Flatulence

Men often joke about this subject but it can be very embarrassing. Flatulence is a sign that the digestive system is not able to handle the breakdown of food. This is because of an overloaded system, poor food combinations, overeating yeasty foods (such as bread, cheese and beer), and also taking high amounts of antibiotics or other forms of medication that wipe out the natural flora of the bowel.

Treatment & prevention program

- Increase fibre in the diet through cereal, psyllium husks and slippery elm bark powder, and by eating more whole fruits such as apples, pears and bananas. Add a teaspoon of psyllium husks to cereal. Slippery elm bark can also be added to cereal or mixed in a glass of water and drunk quickly before it coagulates.

- Take an acidophilus capsule before breakfast and dinner and before bed. This will regenerate the good natural flora in the digestive tract and allow for the easier breakdown of food.

- Don't overeat. Keep the stomach one-third empty after a meal.

- I recommend green tea extract to patients with flatulence. Drinking green tea is good, but the amount that is drunk is usually not enough to improve the condition. In addition to drinking tea, ask for green tea in tablet form and take one tablet three times a day. Reduce to once a day when the condition improves.

- Eat garlic regularly, either as tablets or in its natural clove form as it helps to clean out the bowel.

- Try charcoal tablets – one 300 mg tablet, three times a day between meals – they have been very beneficial for some patients.

- Drink organic peppermint tea three times a day.

✳The liver

Many of the men who come to see me in my practice ask how they can maintain a healthier liver. Many have seen a doctor and have had liver tests, but no problems have shown in the pathology results. And yet they suspect that their liver is playing up due to some of the symptoms they've been having. Generally these symptoms are yellow whites of the eyes, fatigue, irritability, anger, insomnia, and a feeling of being hung-over or seedy.

✳CASE STUDY

I remember a 36-year-old client coming to see me with very low energy levels, grey to yellow whites of his eyes and nausea. He was also very irritable. His lifestyle was very stressful. He lived on takeaway food, mainly Chinese (highly fatty food), and drank a bottle of wine a day, with a few glasses of spirits and occasionally a beer. He did not exercise and was 6 kg overweight. He was also living close to an industrial area.

When his test came back negative for any viral

hepatitis, I was very surprised but explained to him that the pathology of the liver will only show extreme problems and will never show up a sluggish liver or a congested and moderately toxic liver.

I treated him with St Mary's thistle, one tablet three times a day, and included a daily carrot juice and a litre of water in his diet. I also suggested three healthy meals a day, including fish every second day, three to four vegetables in a sandwich for lunch, and steamed vegetables in the evenings with legumes, fish, chicken or lean red meat. Coffee was limited to one a day after breakfast and I suggested he drink no alcohol for six weeks. If he really craved a drink I allowed a gin and tonic in the evening.

On the second visit (four weeks later) he was feeling so much better and I introduced two vitamin B tablets a day, along with two fish oil tablets to assist the detoxification of his liver.

I saw him eight weeks later and the whites of his eyes had returned to their true white colour. His energy levels were 80 per cent better and he was pleased that he had been able to go to gym three times a week because he felt so much healthier. He has now gone back to drinking alcohol but paces himself and continues to take one tablet of St Mary's thistle daily as a preventative for a healthier liver as well as one vitamin B and two fish oil tablets.

The liver is the most overworked organ of the body as it is truly the filter system for all drugs, chemicals, bacteria, hormones, alcohol and any other miscellaneous toxins that come into our bodies. The liver also carries out the major function of keeping blood fats normalised, so it plays an important role in controlling cholesterol (both HDL and LDL). The liver also helps to synthesise and normalise the proteins in our blood. It also manufactures bile to assist in the breakdown of fats. Lastly, the liver has a huge role to play in synthesising and storing glycogen. This is a starchy substance that acts as a store for glucose. If there are inadequate stores, then low blood sugar results, causing tiredness and irritability, and if not checked this can lead to diabetes later in life.

Diseases of the liver may affect or compromise one or all of the above functions.

If you have been travelling, particularly in under-developed countries, ask your doctor to do a blood test to check for viral infection, which can affect the liver and cause hepatitis. Acute hepatitis is usually caused by a virus, but the overuse of drugs and alcohol, and exposure to liver toxins can also cause this disease.

Treatment & prevention program

Dietary changes are a must to take the load off the liver.

- Eliminate fatty foods, alcohol, recreational drugs, red meat, cheese, takeaway food, smoking and fizzy drinks containing colouring and preservatives.

- Refer to the diet for health and vitality (see chapter 12) and include the following juices daily for six weeks: two raw fruit and vegetable juices, particularly freshly squeezed orange and pineapple with a touch of ginger. Also try carrot, beetroot, celery with a touch of spinach and ginger. (You may also like to refer to the liver chapter in my book *Detox*.)

❖ Drink lots of filtered water throughout the day, at least one to two litres. (Do not use tap water.)

❖ Drink herbal teas during the day, such as peppermint or my Triple E or Summer Delight. Dandelion root tea is also great for the liver. Limit coffee to one a day or none at all for six weeks.

❖ Stop alcohol for at least six weeks.

❖ Exercise three times a week.

Supplements

❖ St Mary's thistle (*Silybum marianum*) is great for the liver. This herb assists regeneration of the liver cells and also has a unique ability to protect the liver against toxins. I always advise men to take this herb if they are drinking alcohol on a daily basis, or if they are taking recreational drugs. Take one tablet two to three times a day until the liver symptoms are better and you have more energy and vitality.

▓ A complex vitamin B tablet once daily.

▓ A broad spectrum anti-oxidant to help eliminate free radical
damage.

▓ Two omega 3 and 6 oil tablets a day.

▓ A herbalist can make up the following liver tonic.
  • St Mary's thistle 30%
  • Dandelion root 20%
  • Globe artichoke 20%
  • *Bupleurum falcatum* 10%
  • Liquorice 10%
  • Peppermint 10%
Take one teaspoon twice a day, or three times a day if possible,
in a glass of water. I advise my clients to stay on the tonic for
at least six weeks and preferably twelve weeks to see the
positive results. Note: With viral hepatitis a tonic may be
needed for three to six months.

If your consumption of alcohol has risen, take one
teaspoon of the tonic for two to three weeks after excessive

drinking. I also prescribe a liver tonic for those men who
have stopped smoking and using recreational drugs, to help
their body remove any remaining toxins.

✳Bad breath

Bad breath is usually related to a digestive problem and indicates
that your diet may need to be changed.

Treatment & prevention program

- Avoid fermented foods for six weeks, including cheese,
  alcohol, refined sugar, vinegar, sweets and chocolate.

- Take a digestive enzyme tablet at each meal. Enzymes assist
  the breakdown of foods in the stomach therefore allowing
  better digestion and less fermentation.

- Have regular dental check-ups.

✄ Ensure regular bowel movements (once a day) by including fibre in your diet. I suggest a bowl of cereal each morning with the addition of psyllium husks.

If the problem continues, then take a breath test with your doctor to establish whether you have *Helicobacter pylori*, a bacteria that lives in the stomach and can cause ulcers long term (see page 16).

✳ Gout

Gout, an inflammation of the joints of the feet and hands, particularly affecting the big toe, can be extremely painful. It can come on suddenly, even without a family history of the disease. It is caused by a build-up of uric acid in the system, and many men think that they have just injured their toe until the problem is properly diagnosed. (A blood test can be taken to check uric acid levels.)

Gout often appears after men have binged on rich foods, alcohol – especially red and white wine, cheese and rich sauces.

Christmas time or party time can often bring about an attack, especially when accompanied by low water intake.

Treatment & prevention program

❋ Drink a large glass of water every hour.

❋ Place your foot or hand into a bucket of warm water with a cup of Epsom salts and soak for 20 minutes three times a day. The salts draw out uric acid from the affected area.

❋ Take a teaspoon of fluid extract or tincture of nettle three to four times a day until better. This herb has a great history of assisting gout, going back to the kings and queens of the Middle Ages after they had wined and dined on rich meats and wines. Continue with one teaspoon of nettle in a glass of water once a day as a preventative.

2
Weight

Australian men have been getting fatter over the past ten years. The National Health Survey, carried out by the Australian Bureau of Statistics in 2001, found that 58 per cent of males surveyed were classified as overweight or obese based on their body mass index (BMI). Interestingly, only 30 per cent of males assessed themselves as overweight, indicating a significant gap between perception and reality. These statistics reflect the fact that many men are eating too much of the wrong foods, not exercising enough and are too lazy to change bad habits.

The rule of thumb is this: a man's fat should not exceed 22 per cent of individual body mass. If body fat is measured in excess of this, an individual is classified as obese. Obesity or being over-weight has a detrimental effect on your quality of life. Your susceptibility to heart disease, cancer, diabetes, arthritis, stroke, infertility and other major illnesses is increased dramatically.

Men are particularly prone to accumulating fat around the

abdominal area (the tummy tyre or pot belly), which is regarded as potentially one of the most dangerous forms of obesity. Not only can this be dangerous for your health, it can also be uncomfortable and restrictive of your movement.

✳ Weight loss

There are a number of reasons why men gain weight. Overweight and obese men often present with problems that originate from sugar imbalances, usually a direct result of poor eating habits and lack of exercise. This results in high insulin levels (which can lead to type 2 [adult onset] diabetes). Insulin is the substance released by the pancreas to keep blood sugar levels constant and within the normal range. Eating too many starchy and sugary foods can lead to surges in insulin, which affect the body's ability to burn off fat: high insulin levels suppress the production of the hormone glucagon, which promotes the burning of fat. After a period of time, the body can lose its sensitivity to insulin, which consequently leads to an increase in fat storage. In simple terms, by eating unrefined foods such as fresh fruit and vegetables, organic meat, fish and legumes, and unprocessed grains, you will help your body to maintain regular blood sugar levels, which in turn helps reduce excess fat, increases energy, aids concentration and helps maintain weight within a healthy range.

The culture of Western society does little to promote healthy habits: we have fast food chains as well as the sophisticated technology of television and computers. We eat high-fat, high-sugar, low-nutrition food while sitting passively in front of entertainment. Our daily schedules incorporate little exercise or outdoor activity. Many men's diets include a high intake of refined carbohydrates in the form of hamburgers, fried foods, fizzy drinks, chocolates, cakes and biscuits, as well as a large consumption of beer and alcohol, which are loaded with refined sugar. Weight gain slowly creeps up on everyone with this sort of diet and lifestyle.

Ageing in men is also a factor contributing to weight gain. As men age, physical activity often decreases but eating habits remain unchanged. Many older men are practically sedentary but are still consuming the same high calorie diet as they did when they were younger and more active.

Weight gain can also be triggered by some medications (such as cortisone-based medications, especially those used in treating inflammatory diseases such as asthma, irritable bowel syndrome and arthritis). Excessive stress has also been known to result in excessive weight gain, as many men eat for comfort and relaxation in times of high stress.

Treatment & prevention program

The first and most important step in dealing with excessive weight is to cut out the refined sugars/carbohydrates hidden in so many foods. An excellent starting point is to follow the diet for health and vitality (see chapter 12). It is imperative to remember that when cutting out refined carbohydrates in your diet, you must replace them with other foods. Planning ahead for meals and snacks is essential to maintain the diet and stabilise blood sugar levels. Under *no* circumstances should you miss meals. Because sugar levels will decrease with the absence of refined foods and alcohol, you must eat every four hours, even if you are not hungry, to keep your metabolism and your fat burning system working for you.

Exercise also plays a key role in helping to burn excess fat. Exercising before breakfast or before dinner works well. Do something that you enjoy: the main issue is to safely increase your heart rate which will help you to burn fat as well as improve your cardiovascular system. A trainer can monitor this or you can get advice from a gym. It is especially important to have advice if you are over 50 and suffer from any form of heart disease. Walking does not achieve significant fat loss but is best combined with other forms of aerobic exercise for a weight-loss program.

Lowering stress levels is also beneficial, especially when stress is the background trigger for weight gain. Minimising stress at the same time as establishing a healthier approach to diet and exercise will aid long-term success.

Liver detoxification is a great help in the first stages of a diet and exercise program. A detox ensures that the liver filter system is clean and functions well.

In addition to the diet for health and vitality, take note of these dietary changes to aid in weight reduction.

- Unsaturated fats *must not* be eliminated from your diet. These types of fats include fish oils, flaxseed, avocado and olive oil. These oils enhance fat loss.

Fat and cholesterol

Cholesterol is produced primarily in the liver to carry fats around the body. High density lipoprotein (HDL) is the 'good' cholesterol and we need to have higher amounts of this than of low density lipoprotein (LDL), the 'bad' cholesterol, to maintain good health. Fish oil, vegetable oils and exercise will increase your level of HDLs. Eating foods high in cholesterol such as butter, cream, cheese, eggs and meat will increase your LDL level. When it is oxidised in the body, LDL becomes toxic and, if you do not have enough anti-oxidants in your system, LDL becomes even more dangerous, causing a build-up of cholesterol and increasing the risk of heart disease.

Triglycerides also carry fats around the body, but they are only toxic in high doses. A diet high in refined carbohydrates will increase triglycerides. Take fish oil supplements, follow a low-fat diet and exercise regularly to keep triglycerides at an acceptable level.

High-protein diets have become very popular in recent times, but if unrefined carbohydrates are eliminated totally, experience shows weight loss will only occur at the beginning of a diet. On the other hand, an increase in the number and variety of proteins you consume will help you to maintain your energy levels and muscle mass as you lose weight. The best approach is to find a balance between carbohydrates and proteins in your diet.

- Unrefined carbohydrates that should be part of your diet include brown rice; couscous; wholemeal grainy breads; buckwheat; whole potatoes – including the jacket; root vegetables – including pumpkin, parsnip and sweet potato; barley; split peas and legumes. In my experience with male patients, if you adopt a high-protein diet but don't include some wholemeal carbohydrates, your body will just end up craving sweets or you may indulge in extra alcohol in the evenings.

- Vegetables are an essential part of the diet. Not only are they generally low in fat but they protect the body against cancer, heart disease and arthritis. Vegetables should be included two to three times a day with some form of protein. They can be raw or cooked (preferably include both): at least one to two cups for both lunch and dinner.

- Protein snacks every three to four hours stop you from getting hungry and keep your energy up. Examples of this are ketogenic bars or a protein powder (which has no carbohydrate and can be added to a drink); tinned tuna or salmon on rye biscuits; muesli bars (with no added sugar); soup made from chicken and/or beans; a boiled egg on a rye biscuit with salad; or chunky pieces of chicken on thin Lebanese bread.

- A low-fat soy drink with one of the above snacks is also useful when working long hours.

- Fluid intake should be as high as possible by drinking filtered or bottled water – at least 500 ml every few hours.

- Alcohol in the form of campari and soda or vodka and tonic can be drunk instead of beer and wine as they do not have a high sugar content. (You will just get tipsier faster but not gain so much weight!)

- Fruit can be eaten but it is high in sugar and should be kept to a minimum of two to three pieces daily, preferably eaten by itself, with nothing one hour before or after intake.

A suggested menu

Breakfast

* Scrambled eggs with onion, capsicum and tomato; or hard-boiled eggs. Two eggs every second day.

* A protein shake made from skim milk or soy milk and one piece of fruit, with any wholegrain cereal.

* Baked beans on thin multigrain toast (no butter).

* Tinned tuna or salmon or sardines on thin multigrain toast.

Lunch

* Grilled chicken or steak or tuna (fresh or tinned) with a large salad.

- A tin of mixed beans with a large salad.

- Stir-fried chicken or red meat or tofu with a variety of fresh vegetables.

- Thick vegetable and chicken soup with a large salad.

Ideally, your salad should include a green, a red and a white vegetable. For example: green lettuce or spinach or rocket; red capsicum or tomato; potato salad, cucumber or steamed cauliflower.

Dinner

- Grilled fish or tofu or chicken with steamed vegetables (not potato).

- Grilled steak with salad or vegetables.

- One to two cups cooked rice with a protein and vegetables. You can use couscous instead of rice for variety.

Ideally, try to include at least four different vegetables in your meal.

Eggs

Eggs are a great form of protein and, if you do not suffer from high cholesterol, two eggs every second day in your diet are a very good addition. If you are worried about cholesterol, you can make an omelette from the whites only (the yolk has higher cholesterol-forming properties). If you are including a lot of oily fish like salmon, sardines and mackerel in your diet or taking supplements of fish oil, don't be worried about including a breakfast of poached or scrambled eggs twice a week (but without the fatty bacon, of course!).

Supplements

✂ One or two multivitamin tablets twice daily to correct nutritional deficiencies. Lower dose to two tablets in the morning once you have achieved your weight-loss goal.

❋ One teaspoon of combined magnesium and chromium powder three times a day to assist in controlling insulin levels.

❋ A protein powder such as soy or whey protein: one to two teaspoons, three times a day, to boost protein levels. These powders contain very small amounts of carbohydrates and do not hurt the kidneys. They are useful for men with very busy lifestyles who do not have time to prepare snacks in the office and who eat too late in the evening or who exercise heavily.

❋ Two capsules of omega 3 and 6 oil twice a day. If you have high triglyceride or cholesterol levels, take three capsules twice a day.

❋ You may also consider taking an anti-oxidant supplement. If so, make sure it contains chromium, a trace element which helps control sugar cravings; and a nutrient called L-carnitive, which picks up stored fats and carries them to the cell nucleus to be burnt to generate energy. Coenzyme Q10 also assists this process. You could also try the anti-oxidant alpha lipoic acid, which has been proven to lower high levels of insulin. Check with your health store or naturopath for a combination of these nutrients and correct dosages.

Sugar cravings

Ask your naturopath for a herb called *Gymnema sylvestre* in liquid form. Place five to six drops on the tongue when you are craving sugar. This herb, which grows in India and China, is known to stop sugar cravings and has been used in the Ayurvedic system to assist in weight loss and balancing blood sugar levels.

---

*Waistline reduction

Men who eat only one proper meal each day often suffer from a tummy tyre around the waist or what is commonly known in Australian parlance as a 'gut'. The once-a-day men usually consume their meal at night, which is exactly the wrong time to be eating a main meal when trying to lose weight. Food is for energy and we do not need a massive shot of energy before going to sleep. In fact, sleep disturbances in men are common due to this fact.

Add to this the natural process of ageing. As men grow older, their bellies often grow wider while their legs remain quite lean. Just as women have to work on a flatter stomach, so do men. With a bit of diligence and changes in diet and exercise, big bellies can be significantly reduced.

Treatment & prevention program

There are three main culprits that must be eliminated aggressively if you are to succeed in reducing your waistline. The first of these is fat. Remember, fat creates fat. Cut out all saturated fat: fried foods such as chips and fried eggs; fast foods such as hamburgers; and chocolate.

The other two are sugar and yeasty foods. Sugar ferments with yeasty foods in the gut and puffs you up. This is commonly known as the bloated feeling or bloated look. To prevent this, cut out the following.

- All refined sugars in the form of fast foods, sugar in tea and coffee, beer and wine (you can have three to four glasses of alcohol a week while on this program although it's preferable to cut it out completely for six weeks), white breads, desserts, and rich sauces. Spirits such as vodka, campari and scotch have very little sugar or yeast and are preferable to wine when you are trying to lose weight.

- All foods that contain yeast such as bread (buy yeast-free bread for home or use rice as a base instead – refer to the diet for health and vitality, see chapter 12), wine, beer, cheese (particularly yellow cheese and blue vein cheese), and dried fruits (the concentrated sugars in them will bloat you).

Supplements

- Two acidophilus capsules *before* each meal. This is the good bacteria that needs to be in the gut to assist the breakdown of foods, especially if you have overloaded your system with sugar and yeast-filled foods over a long period of time.

All the following supplements should be taken after food.

✖ Two anti-oxidant tablets (consisting of vitamins A, C and E)
  each morning. These tablets will assist in neutralising the free
  radicals in the body.

Free radicals

Free radicals are the nasties formed in the body by
the combination of oxygen and other elements and
molecules from the environment. They attack cell
tissue, causing deterioration of the cell. In fact this
process is often referred to as ageing, but free radical
damage can be slowed down and in many cases
prevented. Exposure to drugs, smoking, chemicals
and pesticides, pollution and heavy metals, and the
effects of poor diet increase the free radicals in our
system.

The good news is that it has now been proved
that vitamins A, C and E, as well as many plants,
herbs, fresh fruits and red wine, have the ability to
neutralise free radical damage and slow down or even

reverse the damaging effects of these nasties. Plants that have anti-oxidant properties are green tea, grape seed, hawthorn berry, schisandra, St Mary's thistle, turmeric, ginkgo, rosemary, sage and ginger.

Herbalists often suggest taking a combination of such herbs depending on where the free radical damage is most likely to occur. For example, extracts of the active ingredient of green tea are useful for those trying to give up smoking; hawthorn berry for those who have cardiovascular problems; ginkgo, schisandra and ginger for those who need an extra boost in circulation to the brain and extremities.

- Two Siberian or Korean ginseng tablets each morning, especially if you are tired.

- One multivitamin (including all the B vitamins, especially folic acid) each morning. This supplement can be continued for as long as you like.

※ The herb gymnema helps to control blood sugar levels and
cravings. Take one tablet two to three times daily.

Continue taking your supplements until you reach your desired
weight. Then take one of each daily to stay healthy and in control.

Exercise

Exercise is a very important component of any waistline reduction
program. I suggest you talk to a trainer who can set you a program
suitable to your age and body size. Make sure you exercise
aerobically three to four times a week either in a gym or by
running, cycling, rowing, etc. Don't forget to stretch before and
after you exercise to avoid injury.

Swimming is fantastic for toning the tummy tyre but some form
of sprint work to bring up the heart rate should also be included.

Men with a tyre will also need to do the dreaded stomach
crunches to really get rid of that tummy – at least 50 to 80 each day. It
may be easier to build up to this number slowly over a period of time.

3

The immune system and allergies

Today's busy lifestyle means that I often see men who are constantly feeling tired and run-down. Consequently they suffer from conditions such as sinusitis, bronchitis and ordinary colds and flus. The more extensive travel undertaken by many business-men in our increasingly globalised world can also have a detrimental effect on the immune system, while the prevalence of chronic conditions such as asthma has also increased in recent years.

I treat many men who have often been on many rounds of antibiotics. They finally come to see me because they are fed up with the continuing symptoms and problems, and often their specialists have given up on them too.

I also see increasing numbers of men suffering from allergies. An allergy is a hypersensitivity to some kind of foreign substance.

Allergies are different to intolerances and always involve the immune system.

There are two major sources of allergies. The first source is airborne particles such as dust mites (found in carpets, bedding, etc.), pollens (occurring mainly in autumn and spring), and mould (often found in older homes where there is dampness). The other source of allergies is certain types of food. Everyone reacts slighty differently to foods but an allergy sufferer will have a particularly strong and negative reaction. The liver is responsible for our reaction to many foods and controls how efficiently we break down fats and any harmful substances we put into our bodies. I recommend taking the load off the immune system by eating a diet low in foods that cause a histamine reaction, such as red and white wine, milk and eggs.

For those who suffer particularly from pollen allergies, eating fewer carbohydrates, such as bread and pasta, six weeks before the change of season sets in can be of great assistance. These dietary changes also boost the immune system to enable it to cope with airborne particles.

CASE STUDY

A man came to see me who complained of tremendous fatigue and nausea from time to time. He also complained of coming down with terrible flu-like symptoms every three to four months which would lay him up for ten days each time.

On investigation, I discovered that he was a full-time painter who used both oil and water-based paints. He never wore any type of mask while painting. On the positive side, his eating habits were excellent as most of his meals were freshly prepared.

I prescribed St Mary's thistle tablets, one after each meal, to protect his liver and restore any damage from toxic paint fumes; one anti-oxidant tablet, three times a day, to work against free radicals in his system; a combined tablet of echinacea, St John's wort and golden seal to boost his immune system; and a garlic tablet three times a day to act as an antibacterial against infection.

To protect against paint fumes, I asked him to wear a mask when using oil paints, and to drink two to three litres of water daily. I also suggested he gargle half a teaspoon of salt in warm water twice daily.

Ideally, he should keep up this treatment for four months and then to lower his doses to half as a preventative measure, as long as he continues to work as a painter.

Once an allergic reaction has been experienced, treatment needs to be quite aggressive and discipline is needed to make the dietary changes and take the recommended herbs and vitamins regularly for at least three months. I advise my patients that this should be done every year until their system becomes stronger. It is important to stimulate the liver when treating allergic complaints, hence the use of anti-oxidants in a tablet or herbal form.

I always include echinacea and vitamin C in an allergy-treatment program and it is amazing to see the symptoms of sinus and hay fever cut by 50 per cent in most cases.

✳Colds, flus, sinus problems and bronchitis

In my private practice I often see men who have become tired and run-down with bronchial problems and the associated excess mucus or phlegm. It is very rare that they take time off work to rest and recuperate. Occasionally they'll make a quick trip to the doctor to obtain an antibiotic, which can work if there is bacterial infection, but unfortunately has no effect on viral infection.

Sinus congestion causes a mucous drip which can be aggravated in times of stress, at changes of season and by airconditioning. Often this mucous drip causes further problems in the bronchial tubes which can then lead to infection and a barking cough. Doctors refer to this as bronchitis or a croupy cough. If there is a wheeze in the lungs it is often referred to as asthma. Sinus problems and hay fever are often the precursors to bronchitis and shallow breathing.

Plane travel also weakens the immune system and, with the changes in air pressure, sinus sufferers can become quite sick. Airborne allergies in spring and autumn and pollution are huge problems which irritate the sinus passageways. Eyes may become sore, red and itchy. Unless the immune system is boosted and certain precautions taken, the antibiotic merry-go-round will continue. Most people are now well aware that taking antibiotics continually can kill bacteria but will also lower the immune system. What's more, many bacterial strains have become immune to antibiotics.

Treatment & prevention program

Diet plays an important role in preventing colds, flus, sinus problems and bronchitis. Foods that enhance the immune system should be highlighted in the diet, while foods that aggravate the sinus passageways (outside the autumn and spring pollens) need to be avoided or eliminated. Your doctor or naturopath can send you for a food allergy test to identify foods or substances that cause aggravation or sensitivity. When preventative medicine is taken, you build up your immunity, and improvement and relief can be quite remarkable.

CASE STUDY

A man aged 55 came to see me suffering from a severe allergic sinus infection every spring and autumn. He said he had been on antibiotics continually for the last ten years and the specialists, after operating several times, told him they could no longer help him. I explained that he would have to stay on an aggressive dose of vitamins and herbs every seasonal change for the rest of his life. In between the attacks he was to take anti-oxidants to assist his immune system.

He has followed my advice assiduously for the last six years and has had no infections or antibiotics in this time. He takes high doses of vitamin C with bioflavonoids every seasonal change, with echinacea to combat infection and euphrasia to assist with the allergic reactions to pollens. He still has some discomfort but classes himself as 70 per cent better.

The four main food products that have been linked to bronchial problems in many men (although not the sole cause) are:

- grains, especially wheat

- dairy products

- refined sugar

- preservatives and other additives (particularly those found in many wines and highly processed foods).

The prevention program I recommend is as follows.

- Cut out dairy products and cheese. Use low-fat milk on cereal if you can't cut out milk or substitute freshly squeezed orange juice. You may like to try rice or soy milk as an alternative. (Soy milk is also excellent for the prostate.)

- Cut right back on wine and beer and try to drink alcohol that has no added preservatives and additives, such as vodka or campari with tonic or soda. For some men, brandy and gin may also be good options, depending on whether you are allergic to any grains (especially important during seasonal changes).

- Include a freshly squeezed orange juice daily and as much citrus fruit as possible, including pineapple.

- Eat two to three pieces of fresh fruit daily.

- Have half a freshly squeezed lemon with warm water and a little honey (if desired) first thing before breakfast or in the evening. This helps soothe mucous conditions.

- Have some fresh salad with your lunch or dinner. The salad should include green leafy vegetables, tomato (for vitamin C) and any other raw vegetables you enjoy.

- Include cooked or steamed vegetables with your lunch or dinner and aim to have at least three different colours: for example, green could be peas, broccoli, lettuce or spinach; orange could be carrot, pumpkin or sweet potato; white could be potato, cauliflower or cabbage.

- Make the following recipe for a traditional tea for colds, flus and fevers that always seems to work wonders. It is safe for anyone over five years of age. Make up a batch of the following dried herbs and spices, to last you a few days:

- 2 tablespoons peppermint
- $^1/_2$ teaspoon ginger
- $^1/_2$ teaspoon cinnamon
- a pinch of cayenne powder

Combine, and add one teaspoon to a cup of boiling water. Drink hot with honey every three hours.

If you know there are certain times of the year when you usually get sick – flu in winter, sinus problems in spring – or when you'll be travelling, it is vital that you begin the prevention program at least three to four weeks before that time.

Supplements

* Vitamin C with bioflavonoids (such as rutin and hesperin to assist in strengthening the mucous lining of the nasal areas): take 2000 to 3000 mg in powder or tablet form, twice a day, or more often if symptoms are severe.

▓ Two garlic and horseradish tablets, twice a day (or three times a day if your symptoms are severe). (These tablets can often be found containing another herb, fenugreek, which is also helpful.) A tablet made from echinacea, cat's claw and astragalus will boost the immune system. Take one tablet morning and evening all through winter. Double the dose if you feel a flu coming on. A tonic made from the same herbs is even better.

Astragalus (*Astragalus membranaceus*)

The root of this herb has been used for many hundreds of years in traditional Chinese medicine. It is a well-respected plant as a tonic to assist *qi* (energy) and blood nutrition, particularly for enhancing the immune system related to long-term chronic infections. It is a must in the treatment of chronic fatigue syndrome and is wonderful to use after chemotherapy, surgery and any viral infections. I would also recommend this herb to strengthen immunity if you are travelling in countries where health and hygiene levels are poor.

If using a tonic, include liquorice, elecampane, thyme and a little ginger and peppermint. If you are not using a tonic, take a liquorice capsule in conjunction with the herbal immune booster tablet. Liquorice is a wonderful natural anti-inflammatory for the lungs. It also gives energy to the exhausted adrenal glands that become depleted in times of stress.

- Fresh organic peppermint tea with a little cut fresh ginger or a pinch of ginger powder added to the drink.

Bronchitis

If you have a bronchitic cough, ask a herbalist to include herbs such as hyssop, drosera and wild cherry in your tonic. They are wonderful to clear long-standing coughs when combined with the herbs and spices referred to on page 64. All supplements need to be taken for at least six to eight weeks in the case of bronchitis.

Supplements for hay fever

- Two garlic and horseradish tablets every morning and evening.

- Vitamin C with bioflavonoids (500 mg of each) in tablet or powder form in the morning and evening.

- A herb called euphrasia (eyebright) is excellent for treating hay fever. Take one or two tablets three times a day if highly allergic to pollens and grasses. It will dry up a runny nose and watery eyes as well as helping continual sneezing. This herb is also helpful if you work in an airconditioned environment and suffer from the symptoms above.

✳ Asthma

Asthma is a respiratory condition that can be a reaction to certain triggers which narrow the airways. The most common symptoms are difficulty breathing, shortness of breath, tightness in the chest, and coughing and wheezing, particularly at night. Asthma has become more and more common in Australia over the last few years; current statistics indicate that one in ten adults has asthma. There is currently no cure for asthma but it can be managed.

Many asthmatics are allergic to pollens, moulds and grasses and it is therefore important to build up the immune system. Wheat, yeast and dairy products can also be common triggers for shortness of breath. You can ask your doctor or naturopath for a food allergy test to see if there are particular foods which aggravate symptoms.

Treatment & prevention program

Many sufferers of asthma are aware of major triggers; exercise, cigarette smoke, air-conditioning, food allergens, dust mites, pollens and seasonal changes are external factors that asthmatics can control in their daily living.

Simple strategies such as replacing carpets and curtains with floor boards and blinds in your house can be of great benefit. Check the trees and plants in your garden to see if any have high airborne pollens (privet trees are often an aggravation). Use eucalyptus oil burners in your home to clear the air and always use allergy-free cleaning fluids.

Mucus-forming foods such as dairy products (including cream and ice cream), white pasta, white breads, cakes and chocolate must be cut down by 70 per cent. Fresh citrus fruit daily is essential as are three or four different kinds of vegetables.

Supplements

Continue on the prescribed medicine from your doctor and add the following supplements.

- A teaspoon of liquid echinacea twice a day or three to four tablets daily. Taken during seasonal changes and winter, this helps to prevent the onset of upper respiratory problems.

- Magnesium in powder form: take one teaspoon, twice a day. If you can only obtain tablets then take one 500 mg tablet twice a day. Magnesium assists in relaxing the muscles.

- Vitamin C and bioflavonoids in tablet or powder form: 500 mg of each, twice a day.

- A herbal tonic made from equal parts of echinacea, euphrasia, liquorice, thyme, astragalus and peppermint: one teaspoon two or three times a day.

- Coenzyme Q10 – an anti-oxidant that is very useful for treating asthma and emphysema. I suggest 60 to 90 mg, twice a day. It combats damage caused by free radicals, especially if you have been taking long-term medication for asthma. It's also a must for smokers or those who have smoked in the past.

Sinusitis

Recent research has found a strong link between sinusitis and asthma. I encourage men to raise their natural immunity to this condition through long-term use of echinacea root (not leaves) and 3000 mg daily of vitamin C with bioflavonoids. A regular throat gargle made from echinacea and the herb propolis is excellent to prevent a nasal drip.

✳ Travel and the immune system

For those who suffer sinus and bronchial problems, travel can severely affect the immune system, causing an outbreak of symptoms. If you suffer from continual colds and flu when you travel or return from travel, this probably means that your immune system is fighting a virus or bacterial bug picked up on the plane or in the country you are visiting. Over the last few years, I have treated an increasing number of men with these types of complaints, most of whom find themselves doing significant amounts of travel.

To cope with the impact travel has on the immune system, I recommend that you follow the prevention program for sinus problems and bronchitis (see pages 60–64). Be sure to take your supplements away with you, even if your schedule only allows you the time to take them once a day, preferably in the morning after breakfast.

CASE STUDY

A 42-year-old man, a film producer, came to see me because he was suffering continual colds and flus. He was run-down and slightly depressed and lacking vitality. His work demanded that he travel frequently to Asia and the USA. I prescribed a combination tablet of plant extracts with active ingredients against bacterial infections. The tablet included astragalus, echinacea and Siberian ginseng. I also prescribed an anti-oxidant high in vitamins A, C and E to combat free radical damage and to help his sleep patterns during time changes. A calcium tablet in the evening before bed also helped; and I asked him to take melatonin during plane travel and for a week after travel to a different time zone.

On the second visit he was much better, and we addressed some of the dietary changes he could make to improve his fitness during travel (see the diet for health and vitality, chapter 12). I suggested he continue taking his supplements for six months and added co-enzyme Q10 to combat fatigue after long-term viruses.

He is also now more aware of hydrating his body with ten or more glasses of water per day.

Supplements

The following supplements have helped many of my clients who travel frequently for business.

- An immune system tablet consisting of vitamin C and bioflavonoids plus other herbs such as cat's claw, echinacea and astragalus. These are available from your local health store or naturopath.

- One vitamin B complex tablet per day with at least 50 to 100 mg of each of the B vitamins.

- A 100 mg capsule of coenzyme Q10 once or twice a day.

✳ Exhaustion

Many men who consult me have complained of constant fatigue but do not want to discuss this with their family, friends or work mates. They struggle through each day, but they often think there is nothing they can do about it and reject the idea of seeing a doctor for this so-called minor complaint.

After much questioning, I often find that the fatigue has come about through continuing to work while suffering from the flu, a virus or bout of bronchitis, which all result in a lowered immune system. Men often work through these illnesses, and only later do they realise the effect they've had on their body. Blood tests often don't indicate any specific ailment.

There is very little that the medical profession can offer and it is at this point that a good naturopath can try to restore the rundown state of the body that wasn't given rest and recuperation when needed.

Sometimes after a virus you may never feel properly recovered, and if this continues long term it may be diagnosed as chronic fatigue syndrome. The following supplements should offer relief from exhaustion and chronic fatigue syndrome, and boost the immune system.

Supplements

- Two astragalus or cat's claw (or combination) tablets each morning with breakfast. Continue for six to twelve months.

- Coenzyme Q10 – a high dose of 100–200 mg needs to be taken daily for at least six to twelve months. It is the only natural substance that has been found through testing to revive the body after chronic fatigue. I now encourage men who have long working hours, travel commitments and stress to take this enzyme daily to prevent exhaustion and to give them more vitality and energy.

- An anti-oxidant tablet, two per day.

- One multivitamin B tablet with B12 and folate twice a day.

- One Siberian ginseng tablet twice a day (optional), to help the body cope with stress.

Schisandra (*Schisandra chinensis*)

This herb is vital for enhancing the wellbeing of men. In the Chinese medical system, schisandra is regarded as one of the great anti-oxidant herbs with an amazing ability to detoxify the liver and relieve mental fatigue. As a herbalist, I always include this herb with St Mary's thistle for men who have a high workload and who overload their systems with unhealthy food and alcohol. Check with your herbalist for the most suitable dosage.

*Cold sores

The herpes virus exists in the form of cold sores and genital herpes. It is estimated that one in eight Australians now carry this virus. Both forms can now be treated medically but unfortunately the virus will always live in the nerve tissue and attack when you are run-down or have a lowered immunity.

Cold sores usually appear as a series of blisters grouped in a small area around the lips. The blisters quickly dry to form a scab which then takes several days to heal.

If genital herpes is continually recurring then a course of an anti-viral medication is available from your doctor, which suppresses the virus and relieves the debilitating attacks.

Treatment & prevention program

- The herbs St John's wort and astragalus are excellent taken long term to prevent attacks. These herbs act as an anti-viral protection and have been shown in trial cases to reduce the regularity of attacks.

- Take two vitamin B complex tablets twice a day.

✳ Shingles

Shingles is part of the herpes zoster family and is an acute viral infection of the central nervous system where small blisters break out over the line of nerve tissue, generally in the rib cage area or sometimes other parts of the body.

An attack is often related to high stress levels. Although the virus lives in the nerve tissue for a lifetime, many sufferers rarely have an attack, but if attacks are frequent, there are three areas which need to be addressed: stress levels, strengthening the immune system, and eating a healthy diet with low alcohol intake. If attacks are very severe, doctors can prescribe medication. You may also consider the use of preventative medicine during and after the attack. Many older people can have shingles after major surgery or when run-down, especially if their immune system is stressed. The pain can be excruciating and painkillers can be taken if needed.

Supplements

The following supplements can be taken both during an attack and as a preventative measure.

- St John's wort (hypericum): take one tablet, three times a day. This is an anti-viral herb that assists in building up the immune system when you are run-down.

- Vitamin C with bioflavonoids: take 1000 mg of each, three times a day.

- Vitamin E: take 400 IU, once a day. You can also use the oil from a capsule to apply to the dry shingles area after the attack has eased.

- B12 and folic acid: take one tablet (400 mg each), three times a day. They are important for cellular repair and will also help with pain management.

- For the elderly, I suggest a combination tablet of echinacea and St John's wort, one a day, to keep your immune system in good health.

- Zinc is an important mineral for boosting immunity. Your naturopath can do a test to check your levels.

- Many of my patients have used an infusion of a combination of five Japanese mushrooms (hakkumokuji, tochukaso, reiishi, shiitake and chorei) instead of the other herbs suggested above. Take 20 drops, three times a day. Even though they are expensive, this combination is brilliant as an anti-viral and can be used once a day long term as a preventative.

Red eyes

Red eyes are often caused by an allergic reaction to spring pollens and also to histamines contained in red wine, in particular. It's a good idea to observe what time of the year you suffer this problem and after which foods or drinks. Record this information. Your naturopath can then choose the appropriate vitamins and herbs to give you.

Treatment & prevention program

- If you have spring allergies, then take at least 1000 mg each of vitamin C and bioflavonoids, twice a day. This will help considerably. Bioflavonoids such as rutin and hesperin strengthen fine broken capillaries in the whites of the eyes.

- Drink a fresh orange juice daily and eat fresh pineapple each day during the spring season.

- Take euphrasia tablets three times a day if sneezing is associated with redness of the eyes.

✳ Snoring

Snoring can have a devastating effect on relationships and the harmony of family life. It should be taken seriously, especially because lack of sleep can cause other major dysfunctions of your system.

Consult a specialist to establish whether sinus passageways are blocked by adenoids or swollen tonsils. Perhaps it is a case of snoring being caused by allergens and seasonal irritants.

These days surgeons are more reluctant to remove adenoids or tonsils than they were some decades ago. However, if these glands are enlarged, it may be the best option. I have seen some patients who have had surgery to remove the offending organs improve their vitality and quality of life enormously.

Treatment & prevention program

If removal of the glands is not an option for you, then there are some naturopathic approaches that can work well.

- Take vitamin C with bioflavonoids regularly. Ensure you have at least 2000 to 3000 mg per day with equal parts vitamin C and bioflavonoids.

- Take two tablets of garlic and horseradish, twice daily after food.

- Sleep with two pillows under your head.

❈ Always sleep on your side, not on your back.

❈ Cut out red and white wine in the evenings as far as possible as the histamine effect of the wine can interfere with breathing passageways.

❈ Use a light nasal spray containing eucalyptus and peppermint oil before bed.

It's also a good idea to have your iron levels checked via a blood test. Many men are eating less red meat these days, but this can result in low iron levels, especially if you also play sport. If your iron levels are low, a supplement needs to be taken to increase the transport of oxygen around the body and to help remove carbon monoxide from the blood.

4
Sexual health

Sexual health is a field of great importance to men, most especially in terms of how it impacts on their emotional health and quality of life. We are fortunate that issues relating to sexual highs and lows are much more in the public domain these days, and there are now many simple ways of dealing with any problems, and avoiding the potential emotional problems that often accompany it, by changing the diet and using natural products.

✳ Low libido

Many of the men who consult me complain that their libido or sexual drive has diminished or that it is not quite as strong as they would like. This is not exclusively an older man's problem, either. I have had male patients as young as 35 who have come to me to help them with this issue.

When a man is young and complains of low sex drive I usually find that the problem is caused by one or more of the following factors: long working hours, unrelenting stress, poor sleeping habits or interrupted sleep (for example, there may be a new baby in the home). Men aged 50 and over may find their testosterone levels dropping due to age – low sex drive and impaired sexual function are often caused by a drop in levels of this hormone. However, age is not necessarily the problem.

Other factors that have a detrimental effect on sexual function include drug use (and, of course, abuse). Taking marijuana for long periods of time has been found to decrease sex drive and sperm count. Cigarette smoking and alcohol have also been found to impair sexual function.

Mostly, men avoid admitting their lack of interest or function to their wife, partner or lover, struggling to cover up the problem with excuses such as fatigue. Sometimes, men can blame their partners, which usually only exacerbates the tension. In my experience, it is wiser to try to explain the problem to your partner so they can make adjustments and assist you to find healthy solutions.

A decrease in sexual function needs to be discussed with your local doctor and a good naturopath who can suggest ways of dealing with this problem.

Case study

A young man of 32 came to see me about his general health. His girlfriend had sent him. On first consultation I found him to be quite hyperactive, highly focussed on his job as a stockbroker and extremely unaware of his daily eating habits. He complained of tiredness and stress but generally felt he was doing quite well. However, his girlfriend said he was difficult to live with. I asked some simple questions, which finally led to their sex life. He was reluctant at first to tell me that at the moment he was quite disinterested in sex. This had never happened to him. When he and his girlfriend did have sex it took him longer than normal to have an erection and during intercourse he could only perform for a much shorter period of time. He was actually very concerned about this.

He told me he was happy with his girlfriend and he

was worried that she seemed disappointed with him, even though she tried to make light of the situation.

I reassured him that these things can be quite normal when a man even as young as him was working long hours and not eating regularly. In fact it seemed that he was living purely off adrenaline and heading straight for a burn out of the adrenals.

I asked him to eat three regular meals each day which included protein, vegetables and fruits. I also asked him if he could manage to cut out alcohol for six weeks. I think that was a huge shock but he agreed. Fortunately he was not a big coffee drinker.

I prescribed the herb tribulus, one tablet three times a day, for the tonic effect this plant has on reproductive organs, and Siberian ginseng, one tablet three times a day, for support to the adrenal glands. I also insisted that he take a multivitamin B for stress and energy.

He came to see me after four weeks on this program. He was pleased with himself. His libido had improved 60 per cent and he said his sex life was greatly improved. He felt much healthier generally and less jittery. I suggested he keep the same dosage of herbs and vitamins for three months and then bring the dose down to one tablet of each daily or until the stress was under control.

Treatment & prevention program

As a first step towards dealing with low libido, I advise you to embark on a general health program which has the benefits of increasing overall health and wellbeing, as well as increasing sex drive and sperm count (see the diet for health and vitality, chapter 12).

You should start by eating three balanced meals per day on a regular basis. You should also drink eight to ten glasses of water or herbal tea per day. Your protein consumption should be increased to help balance the body's sugar levels and stimulate sperm production. Protein assists the process of building new cells, such as sperm.

Proteins to be regularly included in your diet are:

* fish (preferably deep-sea fish, high in omega 3)

* chicken (preferably free-range and/or hormone-free)

- eggs (preferably free-range); two boiled eggs every second day will not affect cholesterol levels

- beans and pulses such as soy beans, baked beans and lentils (in soups or salads)

- low-fat cheese

- tofu

- lean red meat.

Red meat should be limited to three times a week, at most. Fish and legumes are a better option as they also contain specific substances which assist sexual function, such as isoflavones in soy beans and omega 3 oils in deep-sea fish.

Avoid junk food which carries an overload of refined sugars. These sugars generally lower the body's healthy functioning. Such foods include soft drinks; highly processed cakes and biscuits; and fast foods such as hamburgers and fried takeaways, which are notorious for being full of added sugars and preservatives.

A serious commitment must be made to avoid or give up recreational drugs and smoking. Alcohol consumption should be cut right back to no more than two glasses per day.

Supplements

✖ One tribulus tablet three times a day.

✖ Vitamin E: 500 mg per day. If you suffer from high blood pressure, check with your doctor. This vitamin can thin the blood slightly and has been known to initially cause blood pressure to rise; blood pressure then lowers after vitamin E has been taken for a few weeks. It is wise to begin with 100 mg and slowly increase your dosage to 500 mg.

✖ Siberian ginseng: one tablet three times a day. This has been proved to assist physical and mental stamina, particularly when working long hours or under stress.

Tribulus

Commonly known as tribulus, the herb *tribulus terrestris* is greatly prized in the Ayurvedic health system where it has been used for centuries for its aphrodisiac properties and its tonic effect on the urinary tract and the reproductive systems of both men and women.

In recent studies male volunteers were given 750 mg of tribulus for five days. It was found that their level of testosterone increased. Tribulus has a positive effect on stimulating sexual function and has also been found to improve the mobility and rate of movement of sperm, increase ejaculatory quantity, and improve libido.

The standardised extract of the Bulgarian tribulus leaf must be used. Many products are made from extracts containing the Chinese or Indian tribulus berry, but it is uncertain whether these have the same beneficial effects as the Bulgarian variety. Ask your naturopath or health store assistant to advise if you are unsure.

❊ Vitamin B complex: two tablets each morning to combat general stress and increase energy. Make sure the tablet you choose contains B12 and folic acid which have been found to have the added benefit of preventing heart disease in men.

❊ A herbal tonic made from equal parts of the following:
- damiana (useful if depression is associated with the loss of libido)
- avena (excellent for those who are coming off smoking or recreational drugs as it soothes the nervous system and helps stop the cravings for these substances)
- Siberian or Korean ginseng (increases stamina – Korean ginseng is a little more stimulating and therefore excellent for those who are older)
- liquorice (stimulates the adrenal glands; especially useful for those who play sport and work hard).

Take one teaspoon or 5 ml three times a day or 7 ml twice a day. The tonic needs to be taken with two to three tribulus tablets per day until improvement occurs.

Case study

A young couple in their early thirties came to visit me. The woman had been trying to fall pregnant for two years to no avail. Her reproductive system had been checked and had been given the all clear by the doctors. The man had had his sperm count checked, and while it was quite low, the doctors said it was not too serious.

I found out he worked out at the gym daily. His eating habits were erratic and his protein intake was very deficient. He also said his libido was down. Both he and his wife thought this was normal with busy lifestyles.

He said he was willing to try taking anything to assist his sperm count and libido.

I asked him to take a protein supplement in powder form in a milk shake or water an hour before or after a workout to sustain his energy. Protein intake is an important part of making good quality sperm. I asked him to eat a handful of pumpkin seeds daily for the zinc levels to assist the prostate and his sexual health in general and also to limit beer to every second day. I prescribed tribulus and Siberian ginseng two tablets twice a day for six weeks. I also prescribed an anti-oxidant tablet for free radical damage after exercise: one tablet three times a day. This tablet contained vitamin A, C and E and other herbs with anti-oxidant properties (rosemary, turmeric, St Mary's thistle and ginkgo).

I also asked him to take two of his wife's folate tablets for healthier sperm even though the findings of folate have not been confirmed for sperm count as yet. I believe that this is an essential vitamin not only for women but also for men due to the decreasing rate of meat consumption in our diets. I made sure they were both having a variety of fresh fish, chicken, and legumes regularly with lots of vegetables and fruits. I also included unprocessed grains such as brown rice, couscous, wholemeal grainy breads and a fresh carrot juice daily for its anti-oxidant effects on the liver.

Within three weeks he returned to get more vitamins and herbs. He was ecstatic. He felt his libido had come back and his energy was better than ever before. He had lost some excess flab around the waist and was looking forward to staying on the supplements until his wife fell pregnant. He has been taking the medicines now for six months and his sperm count has increased well into the range of normal.

(Many clients who are on the IVF program come to see me. Herbs and vitamins with a very healthy diet can be of great assistance, but you should always check with your IVF doctor on your intake of natural medication. Most of my clients come to see me before a program or during a break from the program. This is the ideal time to get both parties healthy and to give the appropriate supplements. I have seen amazing results with this approach.)

✳ Impotence

Impotence is defined as the inability to attain or sustain an erection satisfactory for sexual intercourse. It affects 25 per cent of males over the age of 50.

Some of the causes of impotence are long-term alcohol abuse or recreational drug use; hardening of the arteries, usually related to a medical condition such as diabetes or high blood pressure; and accidents or injuries that damage the nerves to the penis. It can also be a psychological or emotional problem – impotence may be a symptom of anxiety or depression or just a result of being overtired or stressed. Sedatives can also have an effect on the ability to sustain an erection.

Treatment & prevention program

Following the diet for health and vitality (see chapter 12) is a good first step to take to deal with the problem of impotence. A healthy diet and regular exercise can help eliminate some of the causes of this condition. If you suspect that emotional problems are the cause, ask your doctor or naturopath to refer you to a respected counsellor.

Supplements

❊ Tribulus (see page 91): two to three tablets a day.

✳ One tablet of *Panax ginseng* once or twice a day, or 3 ml of the liquid once a day. A great tonic for the sexual organs.

✳ *Ginkgo biloba*: one tablet daily to assist peripheral circulation.

✳ One vitamin B complex tablet, for general stress.

✳The prostate gland

The prostate gland is now a common topic of conversation among men. It is a subject that has received an increased level of media attention in the past few years and about which men in general are very concerned. One in ten Australian men will develop prostate cancer and it is now the second most common form of cancer diagnosed after skin cancer in Australia.

The prostate is a small gland whose main job is to make the liquid that carries sperm, hence its unseen effect on men's sexuality. In fact, the nerves that generate erections surround the prostate. It is wrapped around the tube called the urethra which carries urine to the penis. If the prostate is enlarged, the flow of urine is inhibited. This causes a frequent need to urinate, especially in the evening. The urine is passed in small amounts.

If the prostate is enlarged enough, the condition becomes known as prostatitis, which is an inflammation or swelling of the prostate gland. It is often associated with an infection of the gland which can be bacterial or non-bacterial.

Acute prostatitis is caused by a bacterial infection of the gland and usually affects younger men between 25 and 50 years of age. Common symptoms include painful urination, painful ejaculation and flu-like symptoms such as aches and chills. This form of prostatitis can be treated successfully with antibiotics but you can also try using the supplements below for a more natural solution to the problem.

Chronic prostatitis is usually associated with a non-bacterial infection of the gland and occurs most commonly in males over 45 years of age. Common symptoms include painful and frequent urination, particularly at night, painful ejaculation, lower abdominal pain and pain at the base of the penis or along the shaft. If these symptoms are not treated, it can lead to complete obstruction of urination and infection. It is estimated that 60 per cent of males between the ages of 45 and 60 will have an enlarged prostate.

Where prostate cancer is diagnosed, a decision usually needs to be made whether or not to remove the prostate. If it is not removed, but treated, the risk is that further cancer may develop in the body.

The prostate can be monitored, like the breast in women, with regular testing by your local doctor. Many men dread having a rectal examination by the doctor, but it is necessary to ensure that the prostate is not inflamed. It is critical that you realise the importance of regular checks – once a year for those at high risk (i.e. those whose father or brother have had prostate cancer at an early age) or those over 40. A blood test called a PSA (Prostate Specific Antigen) test can also be done.

Treatment & prevention program

All men over the age of 30 should be aware of the benefits of having a healthy diet (see the diet for health and vitality, chapter 12). Foods containing saturated fats, such as fried foods, chocolate and takeaways, should be limited, as should refined carbohydrates such as sugar in alcohol, sweets and cakes. I also recommend that you increase your use of soy products, for example, replace ordinary milk on your cereal with soy milk.

Men aged 40 and over should include the following in their diet:

- Foods that are high in zinc such as oysters, pumpkin seeds, nuts and whole grains (especially sourdough rye bread).

Zinc

The prostate gland needs high amounts of zinc to function. The zinc content of many foods we eat has been reduced by the chemicals and fertilisers used in the soil. A simple zinc taste test can be done by your naturopath to assess your nutritional level of zinc. It is not necessary to supplement with this mineral if your level is within the normal range.

- Foods that protect the prostate such as almonds, sunflower seeds, garlic, onions and shallots (which contain natural sulphur and active ingredients that assist arterial integrity). For example, eat a handful of almonds and pumpkin seeds two to three times a week as a snack.

- Soy products such as soy milk, tofu and tempeh. These are all high in substances called isoflavones that work against prostate cancer.

- Omega 3 and 6 oils – omega 3 is found in oily deep-sea fish such as salmon, cod, mackerel and sardines; omega 6 is found in flaxseed oil and evening primrose oil.

- Fresh filtered water – at least eight to ten glasses per day. This is essential to flush the urethra, the tube that extends from the bladder to the exterior. This is especially important after heavy alcohol intake.

- Cranberry juice. This assists the functioning of the bladder and prevents the build-up of bacteria in the bladder tubes. Only buy the best quality from your local health store and dilute with water.

- Reduce coffee and sugar intake.

Supplements

❖ A combined omega 3 and 6 oil capsule: two to four capsules daily. This is wonderful not only for the prostate but it has also been shown to decrease cholesterol levels and prevent heart disease in men.

❖ One B-complex tablet with 50–100 mg folate daily. Folate has been found to protect against prostate cancer. Folate is also found in abundance in green leafy vegetables.

The following supplements are useful specifically for treating prostatitis.

❖ Saw palmetto (*Serenoa repens*): one tablet after every meal (three times a day) until better, then one per day as a preventative measure. This herb is brilliant for treating prostatitis. If a lowered sex drive accompanies the prostate problem, include tribulus – two to three capsules daily (see page 91).

- Liquid zinc, 1 ml diluted in 100 ml of water. Your naturopath may recommend a higher dose. If you prefer taking tablets, take zinc sulphate, 100 mg per day. One dozen oysters contain around 120 mg of elemental zinc.

- Two capsules twice daily of omega 3 and 6 oils.

- One tablet after each meal or a teaspoon twice a day in water of vitamin C and bioflavonoids (500 mg of each). This acts as an anti-oxidant, particularly where there is inflammation or an infection.

- One tablet of *Panax ginseng* twice daily or 3 ml of the liquid tincture daily is recommended. This herb helps the body to deal with stress, both physical and mental. In Chinese medicine ginseng has long-term beneficial effects on the sexual organs.

- A herbal tonic made from equal parts of: nettle, crateva, willow bark, cornsilk and Siberian ginseng (include ginseng only if not taking *Panax ginseng* tablets above). Take one teaspoon twice a day until the condition improves. This tonic, which assists the flow of urine, should be taken in conjunction with all the supplements in this section, particularly saw palmetto.

If you have prostate cancer, you can see a naturopath about complementary therapies to run alongside your essential medical program. This can be discussed with your doctor.

5

A healthy heart

Heart disease kills more people in the Western world than almost all other diseases together, including cancer. The astonishing irony is that heart disease is the most easily preventable disease, yet the most serious of our time.

I know some men have the attitude that, when it comes to heart health, it's a question of 'When my time's up, my time's up'. Unfortunately, they haven't thought about the possibility of surviving a heart attack or stroke. Survivors often have a severely impaired quality of life. Consider life in a wheelchair or with a speech impediment. Not a great prospect for the rest of your years on earth!

There is a lot we now know about preventative health in relation to heart disease and yet there is rarely a concerted effort or plan to incorporate it into our lifestyle. Sadly, that often happens after the event. For example, we know from the education of the 80s and 90s that exercise is imperative. Exercise, along with a diet low in saturated fat, is a great preventative.

In my clinical experience it is often just a matter of inspiring men to follow an easy daily guide. This keeps their hearts ticking along nicely with the confidence that they are doing all in their power to lower their risk of disease before it happens. It is not necessary to eliminate all the good things in life. It is a question, as always, of balance.

Exercise and relaxation

Exercise is essential for the cardiovascular system and keeps cells oxygenated. It is important to stick to an organised exercise program three to four times a week for at least an hour. Walking daily (fast) is a good start. Those who have had a heart problem should wear a heart monitor when exercising. In fact, if you have not exercised for quite some time, ask a professional at your local gym to check out your fitness level and monitor your heart rate before you start a program.

It's not unusual to hear of men who haven't exercised for some time who go out to the tennis court or the golfing fairway and suffer a heart attack. The danger is in straining the heart too much initially through overexertion. Play safe and build your exercise program gradually. Don't go at it unprepared.

As well as incorporating exercise into your life, you should also find a form of relaxation that you really enjoy. Make sure you take regular holidays, relax daily through meditation, reading or walking or whatever you find slows down your heart rate and empties your brain of unwanted thoughts.

If you are unhappy, or have experienced trauma of any kind through a divorce, break-up, death or separation of any kind, this may be the time for you to take stock of your life. This is especially important if high blood pressure, cholesterol, heart palpitations and anxiety are present.

Make sure you are assessed regularly by your doctor, and include all checks related to the heart and cholesterol. Remember, prevention is much better than fatality.

Treatment & prevention program

The following is a suggested treatment and prevention program for those concerned about the health of their heart. It is also suitable for those who have suffered a heart attack or stroke. I would advise anyone who falls into the latter category to ask your naturopath and medical doctor to confirm the dosages for any supplementation.

To avoid heart problems, it is best to adopt a healthy lifestyle. Smoking, being overweight, drinking too much alcohol and caffeine, eating fatty foods, living a sedentary life, and having high stress levels are all factors which can contribute to heart problems and should be eliminated or reduced.

- Eliminate foods containing saturated fat from your diet, such as butter, ice-cream and fried foods.

- Reduce refined sugars in your diet such as the sugars present in beer and wine, tea, coffee, cakes, biscuits and confectionery. (Note: a high consumption of sugars and carbohydrates tends to bring up triglyceride and cholesterol levels).

> ### Red wine
>
> Red wine is high in flavonoids, which are classed as an anti-oxidant. Moderate drinking of red wine is fine, but remember it contains alcohol which, in high doses, is not useful for the liver or the cardiovascular system. I suggest you limit red wine to two glasses every second or third day. (Avoid white wine. It does not contain these helpful substances and is detrimental to those who suffer gastric ulcers, irritable bowel or an acid stomach.)

- Make sure you add to your diet on a regular basis (daily wherever possible) the following:
  - A serving of deep-sea fish such as cod, salmon, mackerel or sardines (grilled or lightly sautéed in unsaturated oil). Sardines can be used as a snack on toast three to four times a week. Deep-sea fish contain omega 3, which has been found to be essential in encouraging the production of 'good' cholesterol and lowering 'bad' cholesterol.
  - A variety of proteins, including a legume soup (legume

means beans such as those found in minestrone soup),
three times a week. Chicken, red meat (but only two to
three times a week), eggs (two every second day), and the
occasional handful of almonds (not peanuts and brazil
nuts) are also good sources of protein.

- Anti-oxidant fruits and vegetables two to three times a
day. Concentrate on incorporating three colours of
vegetables and fruits daily, including orange (such as
freshly squeezed orange juice, mangoes, peaches, sweet
potato, pumpkin, carrots). A raw carrot juice each day is
ideal. Green vegetables include a green salad, peas,
zucchini and broccoli. White vegetables include
cauliflower, potato, onions and garlic.
- Lots of garlic, onions and shallots. These foods can help
lower blood pressure and cholesterol.
- Plenty of filtered water. Start the day by drinking a large
glass of water at room temperature with the juice of a
quarter of a lemon. For an average-sized man, drink two
litres of water daily. Water can be replaced in part with
juices or herbal tea.
- Some form of fibre once or twice a day to keep the bowel

healthy and cholesterol down. This includes cereals, grainy breads, brown rice and grains such as couscous. I suggest you put a tablespoon of psyllium husks on your cereal daily or in a glass of water as this form of fibre has been shown to assist in lowering cholesterol.

- If you are 45 and heart disease runs in the family, a doctor will often suggest you take half an aspirin daily (make sure you buy the coated aspirin that is not acidic to the stomach lining) to help keep the blood thin and prevent blood clots. Omega 3 and 6 oils have also been shown to assist this. I advise you to discuss the best solutions with your doctor and naturopath.

Supplements

The following supplements are wonderful to help prevent heart disease and stroke.

- One or two omega 3 and 6 oil capsules daily. A higher dose – three capsules twice daily – can help reduce mild cholesterol problems over a period of three to four months.

Omega 3 and 6 oils

I advise most of my male clients to take these wonder oils to reduce their risk of coronary heart disease. Omega 3 oil comes from cold-water fish such as salmon, cod, mackerel, tuna and sardines, and also from flaxseed oil. It is often referred to as high potency marine oil and it contains essential fatty acids. Essential fatty acids are found in high concentrations in the constitutions of Greenland Eskimos. The fact that these individuals have a very low incidence of ischaemic heart disease, despite consuming very high levels of animal fat, has been attributed to their consumption of these oils. They lower serum triglycerides and total cholesterol while increasing the good cholesterol HDL. Omega 6 oils are sourced from evening primrose oil and soy oil.

When buying capsules, the oils should be in a ratio of four to one: that is, four times more omega 6 oils than omega 3 in the capsule.

✽ Vitamin E: one 500 IU tablet per day. This has been shown to
be an outstanding anti-oxidant that assists the healthy
working of the heart. This can be obtained in a combined
tablet form with your omega oils. Check the dose with your
doctor if you already have high blood pressure.

✽ Hawthorn berry: one tablet twice a day. This herb assists mild
to high blood pressure and is an excellent anti-oxidant for the
heart. It also helps dispel fluid retention.

Hawthorn berry

Hawthorn berry contains active ingredients referred
to as flavonoids, including quercetin glycosides and
oligomeric procyanidins. These have been found to
be effective in the treatment of mild heart conditions
and for prevention of angina pectoris, coronary heart
disease, cardiac arrhythmia, hypertension and
arterial degeneration.

❋ Magnesium: two to four 200 mg tablets a day (especially if you are very active). This helps to keep the heart beating at a regular rate. Magnesium is a wonderful mineral for all muscles but especially the largest muscle in the body – the heart.

❋ Coenzyme Q10: 60–100 mg per day is ideal as a preventative; double the dose post-heart attack for a good six months. This is an excellent supplement to help create intracellular energy and vitality. It assists the mitochondria (the actual computer of the cell) in its essential work. This enzyme has been found to be of great help not only in chronic fatigue but also for those in recovery after a heart attack or stroke.

❋ One to two multi-B vitamin tablets (which include B12 and folic acid) per day.

Folic acid (folate)

Recently articles in medical journals have reported how essential folic acid is to prevent cardiovascular disease and Alzheimer's. Clinical evidence now clarifies that low folate levels can cause dementia and arteriosclerosis. A simple blood test by your doctor can check if you have high homocysteine (a toxic amino acid by-product) levels in your blood. A high level would be above 8. If so, it is essential for you to take a therapeutic dose of 5 mg of folic acid, which you can buy from a pharmacy. As a preventative measure (especially for men over 50), you can take 400 mg folic acid with 400 mg B12 (B12 works with folate to keep nerve pathways healthy).

※ One garlic tablet (one which includes the active ingredient allicin) or a clove of crushed garlic daily. In clinical trials, garlic has been shown to reduce fats (lipids) in the blood. It is believed that the real value of garlic is in the prevention of cardiovascular disease. Garlic must be included in any program for lowering cholesterol.

Multivitamins

Some men take a multivitamin tablet as a matter of course each day. It's worth asking your naturopath to check the dosage as often they are far from therapeutic for your needs and lifestyle. Make sure it has all the already listed supplements. If not, then I suggest you take them separately, especially if you are at high risk of heart problems and are not changing your diet. If you travel and tend to eat and drink more on those occasions, then definitely take the supplements recommended in this section to counteract potential problems.

CASE STUDY

A few years ago I had a 38-year-old man consult me. He had suffered a minor stroke which had left him with impaired speech and a slight limp. His lifestyle as a stockbroker in the USA had been fast and furious; he took recreational drugs on the weekends and ate mainly takeaway foods. His alcohol intake was enormous as he entertained at lunch and in the evenings most days.

He told me that his father had survived a heart attack at 55. This young man had never had his cholesterol checked and did very little exercise. While he told me he thought he was too young to have anything wrong with his cardiovascular system, the trend is for younger and younger men to suffer from strokes and heart problems, especially if there are hereditary and lifestyle factors involved.

I recommended high doses of coenzyme Q10 (200 mg daily) and vitamin E (1500 IU daily) as well as two hawthorn berry tablets daily.

When I saw him twelve months later he was 90 per cent better. His attitude towards his lifestyle was quite different and he only wished that he had realised the damage he had been causing his body during preceding years.

6
Stress

Stress is a major contributing factor to many diseases, and can have a negative impact on preventative health and general happiness. Men have an uncanny ability to hide their stress levels, but then drink larger amounts of alcohol, or smoke or take some form of recreational drugs to help them get through stressful times. Many of my clients know how important it is to exercise and get the stress out of their system but they often don't realise how important it is to eat healthy foods within a balanced diet when undergoing high pressure. Taking some form of supplements, even if it is only for a short time, during heavy mental and physical strain can be a lifesaver and stop many complications such as chronic fatigue, adrenal exhaustion and the everyday symptoms of irritability and mood swings.

In this chapter I've offered some simple solutions to utilise in your everyday life. Begin with a dedication to a healthier diet, followed by one or two supplements that I suggest you take for three months. Then see how you feel. The main comment I hear from my male clients who follow this path is that they are not nearly so reactive to stress and they now wake up in the mornings with so much more energy and mental stamina, looking forward to the challenges of the day.

✳ Anxiety and depression

Many men do not admit even to themselves that they are suffering highs and lows or mood swings. They can very effectively ignore continual nagging feelings of depression. Other men admit to me in my clinic that they suffer panic attacks and a feeling of gloom, but would never discuss this with their partner, family or work associates.

I find that vast improvements can often be felt simply by addressing diet. If men do not eat regularly – at least three meals a day – then unstable blood sugar levels can play havoc with the brain. Concentration becomes poor and you can become prone to outbursts of anger. Tension associated with sugar imbalance can build up to unacceptable levels.

The impact of stress on the chemicals in the body is very complicated. Good nutrition is so important, but when a man has a large workload or suffers from long-term stress, taking supplements for three to six months can do wonders. After this period, you may choose to continue taking a preventative dose of the supplements on a daily basis.

Adrenal exhaustion is a common complaint. When overworked and stressed, the adrenal glands (they sit on top of the kidneys) produce an overload of the natural hormones adrenaline and cortisol. The body can accept a certain level of stimulation which keeps you 'revved up', but abnormally high levels over a long period of time can lead to exhaustion, anxiety, depression and a general feeling of complete fatigue.

Cortisol levels can now be checked by a blood test. If they are abnormally high, they tend to suppress the feel-good hormone serotonin. This can lead to both moderate and severe forms of depression. Cortisol levels should be higher in the mornings and lower in the evenings. Siberian ginseng definitely assists the adrenals to withstand stress and pressure. In my practice I recommend this herb to men who are working long hours and to those who are recovering from surgery or trauma of any kind.

Neurotransmitters in the brain can also affect your stress levels. The brain is a highly complicated organ and selective in its requirements. Poor diet, smoking, drugs, alcohol and everyday stress all affect the chemical reactions in the brain.

Recent research now recognises how essential B12 and folic acid are for depression (as well as for heart conditions and Alzheimer's). It has also been found that high levels of homocysteine (see page 115) cause the lowering of blood levels of a substance referred to as SAMMe (s-adenosylmethionine – a derivative of the amino acid methionine). It is vital to take SAMMe supplements if you suffer from depression, panic attacks and insomnia related to depression. It is usually mixed with B12 and folic acid which have been found to increase the effects of SAMMe.

Another substance that works on depression is 5-hydrozy-tryptophan, nicknamed 5-HTP. This substance is found naturally in the body and forms the building blocks for the feel-good hormone serotonin. A supplement of 200 mg a day is ideal, although often you will find this mixed in a formula with SAMMe. Tryptophan is also found in the following foods, so make sure you eat plenty of these in your diet; it's very high in pumpkin (578 mg per 100 gm), sunflower seeds, cheese, meats, turkey and peanuts.

Hypericum (St John's wort) can also be used to treat depression. It's mainly known for its use in cases of mild depression. Note: If you choose to use a 5-HTP supplement, do not use hypericum with it as you may become too euphoric.

Treatment & prevention program

- For men who are suffering anxiety or depression, the diet for health and vitality (see chapter 12) is an essential first step.

- Drinking water regularly is vital, preferably two litres a day.

- Cut down on the intake of alcohol, which can act as a depressant.

- Increase exercise which has been proved to stimulate the production of endorphins, the 'feel-good' hormones in our systems.

Supplements

- A high dose B multivitamin tablet (containing 100 mg of the main B vitamins and 50–100 mg of folate): two tablets in the morning and two in the afternoon for the first month; then continue taking two each morning.

- SAMMe is an extremely important supplement to take if you suffer from depression or panic attacks (see page 124). It's usually mixed with B12 and folic acid in tablet form: take one tablet morning and evening.

- 200 mg magnesium tablet twice daily, or more frequently if very anxious. Magnesium is vital as a relaxant to muscle tissue, especially in situations of stress.

- One tablet of hypericum (St John's wort) twice a day of the standardised extract, or as prescribed. This can be used as an alternative to SAMMe (but I advise not to use them together).

- One tablet of combined *Ginkgo biloba* and bacopa three times a day, for stress and general exhaustion. These herbs alleviate mental and physical fatigue, and improve concentration.

- One Siberian ginseng tablet twice daily if under stress. Take for three months only then stop for six weeks.

If depression and anxiety continue to be a problem, I advise my male patients to discuss with their doctors the possibility of seeking some form of emotional support and counselling. This is especially important when men are going through a separation, divorce or 'change in life'.

Panic attacks

A number of men I have treated admit to having some form of anxiety attack or panic attack that comes upon them suddenly, even when relaxing. The best way of dealing with this type of attack is to slow down your breathing. Take ten deep breaths, holding each breath for 10 seconds. (See also meditation on page 158.) This process increases carbon dioxide in the blood, which will allow the available oxygen to be released into the body's cells and the natural balance to be restored. It is this imbalance that can cause anxiety to spiral into panic.

Treatment & prevention program

❋ Avoid coffee, stimulants and hot, spicy food.

Supplements

❋ Magnesium supplements, 1000 mg daily, to help normalise the rhythm of the heart and relax the muscles from daily stress.

❋ St John's wort: start with two tablets twice a day and then cut the dose by half as you improve. This has been shown to be very helpful in counteracting panic attacks. Taken long term, this herb not only alleviates anxiety but also eases the often detrimental effects of anxiety attacks after a virus.

❊ A herb called passion flower mixed with a Chinese herb called *Zizphus jujuba* can assist with anxiety attacks if they are not associated with depression. Take one or two tablets after each meal until your condition improves, then reduce to one a day.

❊ B12 and folic acid in a vitamin B formula: one tablet a day. If attacks are very severe then take a supplement which also includes SAMMe. Two tablets twice daily until better, then two every morning as a preventative measure.

✳Insomnia

There are many reasons why men are often restless sleepers. Poor diet, eating late at night, stress, anxiety and caffeine can all affect sleep patterns. Sinus problems (blocked breathing passageways), swollen tonsils and adenoids can also play a part in sleep apnoea and snoring, which can cause men to wake up tired each morning.

If you have a history of sinus problems, then this needs to be addressed with your medical doctor (see also chapter 3).

Treatment & prevention program

✂ Follow the diet for health and vitality (see chapter 12) to
address dietary issues.

Supplements

The following supplements can assist men to establish much
healthier sleep patterns. I suggest you start with a calcium
supplement if you suffer from mild insomnia. Depending on the
results, you may then work through the other supplements and see
what is right for you, depending on the reasons for your insomnia.

✂ Calcium: take a 500–1000 mg calcium tablet before bed and
another if you awaken in the middle of the night. Many of my
clients have great success with this if taken with a cup of
chamomile tea.

✂ Passion flower rapidly reduces stress and relaxes the nervous
system. Take two tablets before bed for at least three to four
weeks and then when required.

* *Zizphus jujuba*, a Chinese herb, calms the nervous system. Take 3 mg before bed. Herbalists often mix this with passion flower, skullcap and hops.

* One to two SAMMe tablets three times a day. This has been found to be useful, especially if your insomnia is related to depression or frequent jet lag.

* Melatonin is a hormone that is excellent for jet lag and those who travel extensively. It is produced naturally in the brain during deep sleep and REM sleep. Doses of 3 mg can be obtained from pharmacies in the USA but is not yet available in Australia, where it is still in the process of being approved. Sunlight stimulates the production of this hormone naturally, which is why it is always recommended that travellers try to expose themselves to sunlight when changing time zones.

* Mexican valerian has helped some of my clients to sleep when under high pressure at work. This herb should be taken 15 minutes before sleeping: two tablets 20 minutes before bed. You may wish to use this herb when travelling.

7

Joints

✳

✳ Rheumatoid arthritis

Arthritis is the word used to describe inflammation of the joints. It is often described as an auto-immune disease as it relates to the system within the body which produces antibodies.

In the modern medical approach to arthritis, anti-inflammatory drugs are used which are either steroidal or non-steroidal. Unfortunately joint disease is poorly understood and the treatments have not advanced for a long time. Hopefully more research into the causes and the cure of joint diseases will be done over the next few years.

Naturopathic approaches are certainly worth trying. They may not cure the disease but they can certainly relieve much of the discomfort and slow down the debilitating symptoms. Diet plays a huge role in controlling the symptoms and some plant medicine and nutritional supplements can be very beneficial.

My father, who had severe arthritis in his knees, was always joking about the fact that there was no cure for joint problems, and he was very disturbed that the anti-inflammatories he was prescribed were upsetting his stomach, which is a very common side effect. Just by increasing his intake of water each day (elderly people tend to be dehydrated because they don't consume enough water daily) and including some vitamins helped him.

In all treatment of joint problems, solutions must be looked upon as long-term: a lifestyle change and a commitment to taking the supplements regularly to stop degeneration and further damage to the immune system are essential.

Treatment & prevention program

✂ Follow the diet for health and vitality (see chapter 12). This is imperative. All junk food, white sugar and white flour products must be eliminated. Foods that nourish joints are those containing omega 3 and 6 oils, such as deep-sea fish, flaxseed oil, and vitamin E in avocados and wheatgerm oils.

- Eat high-quality proteins such as legumes, eggs and white meat, which are more suitable than red meat, as one of the waste products from digestion of red meat is uric acid which can aggravate joints.

- Drink celery juice daily as it assists the balance of potassium and sodium being carried to the joints. It can be mixed with carrot juice.

- Avoid acidic foods such as rich sauces, white wine, white vinegar, and some fruits such as oranges, strawberries and other berries which can aggravate joint problems. It is best to stay off these foods for six weeks and introduce them back into your diet slowly and see if they affect your level of joint pain in certain quantities.

- Drink lots of pure, filtered water.

- Encourage mobility of the joints through exercise such as water exercises and walking. Running is very aggravating to any joint, especially on a hard surface.

Supplements

▓ Two omega 3 and 6 oil capsules twice daily. It lubricates joints. Double the dose if in severe pain.

▓ One glass of celery juice daily or two celery tablets daily. For taste and health, mix with carrot juice.

▓ Two tablets of the standardised extract of boswellia twice daily or one tablet daily as a preventative. Boswellia, which acts as a natural anti-inflammatory, is excellent for arthritis (and also for inflammation of the bowel). There is often a link between inflammation of the bowel and arthritis. You may find this herb mixed with ginger and turmeric (both natural anti-inflammatories).

▓ One or two ginger capsules three times a day. Ginger tablets have relieved many joint problems because they stimulate the circulation. They are especially useful for those in cold countries, to assist mobility. In fact they are very useful when skiing or participating in water sports in cold water.

▓ Glucosamine sulfate (see page 135): one tablet two to three times a day.

▓ I have made many wonderful tonics for arthritis using traditional herbs, and if the client stays on these daily over the winter period, when joints seem to be at their worst, the aches and pains are kept under control without the long-term effects of anti-inflammatories. The following tonic is recommended.

- Equal parts of celery, dandelion, prickly ash, boswellia (you can also take this herb separately as a tablet for better results), willow bark, devil's claw, liquorice, ginger and astragalus (which helps the immune system in chronic conditions). Take one teaspoon in water twice daily.

▓ A liniment containing the Chinese herbs kadsura, pothos and curcuma, and menthol, camphor and some wintergreen oil. These are available at your health store. Rub on the affected area.

✳Sports injuries

Usually I leave sports injuries to a chiropractor or sports medicine practitioner, but I have found some nutritional supplements to be quite miraculous in healing torn ligaments and bruised muscle tissue. They are definitely worth using as a preventative in smaller doses if you exercise regularly and suffer from old injuries to your joints from sport.

Training and stress often deplete intra-cellular magnesium, which regulates the secretions of the hormone cortisol from the adrenal glands. If you suffer disturbances in your magnesium levels, which is often the case when doing heavy exercise, then your cortisol levels are also affected which can lead to some forms of depression and anxiety.

Supplements

※ Magnesium is essential for those who have a build-up of lactic acid in muscle tissue from sport, resulting in cramping. It can be taken in an electrolyte drink, powder or tablet form.

Take at least 400–800 mg daily depending on the severity of the problem.

�֎ One teaspoon of sea salt in a glass of water on acute cramping. In most cases, the cramping will disappear instantly. If you are sweating a lot, you will lose sodium. Many men follow low-salt diets but it is essential to use sea salt daily on your food, preferably half a teaspoon each day.

✖ Glucosamine sulfate is a natural substance (a major constituent of cartilage) that has worked wonders in regenerating ligaments and any form of connective tissue. It assists all the ball and socket joints. I prescribe this for any arthritic and rheumatic problem. Take a 500 mg tablet three times a day. This is the recommended dose to see results over a period of two to three months. Reduce the dose as the condition improves. Often these tablets contain a small amount of copper and manganese with vitamin C and zinc for absorption and added effectiveness.

✖ Injuries often occur because protein is not replaced within half an hour of heavy exercise. I suggest you drink a protein powder after exercise. This can be mixed and taken to work or the gym and drunk after your workout. It will repair and replace essential mineral chelates. You may also wish to use an electrolyte drink if you are training heavily and working long hours. These minerals are essential if you sweat a lot and feel continually tired.

- An anti-oxidant tablet containing vitamins A, C and E or anti-oxidant herbs is essential for those who exercise frequently and/or heavily. Take two tablets two to three times a day. They help prevent free radical damage to cell tissue.

- Boswellia is wonderful for those who suffer from any inflammation in joints and muscle tissue. This herb can be introduced as a supplement if you have joint problems in conjunction with irritable bowel or an acidic system. Take two tablets a day in the morning after breakfast. Always buy a tablet which provides you with a standardised extract (check the label).

⁜   Turmeric has been found to be useful if taken acutely: two
    tablets every hour, then three times a day as you improve.

This program is also very useful for those coming off anti-
inflammatory drugs because these supplements regenerate and
rebuild. They are truly remarkable.

Muscle spasms

If you suffer from muscle spasms and pain following
exercise, you may find that two to three magnesium
and calcium tablets (in a 2:1 ratio) three times a day
helps to relax spasms and ease pain. Alternatively
you can often buy a magnesium powder with
chromium which works faster than the tablets.
Take one heaped teaspoon every three hours. Use
a liniment for the relief of injuries to the muscle.

8

Skin

Many men are concerned about their skin and how it affects the way they look, even if this is not the main reason they come to see me. Even though they seem to have fewer problems than women, they still worry about conditions such as redness of the skin, dermatitis and psoriasis.

Many men find that creams do not work very well or only provide a temporary solution.

Skin problems may appear seasonally, in spring and autumn, when allergies affect the immune system (see chapter 3). Stress is also a major contributing factor to skin problems, and stress often leads to poor eating habits and an increase in the use of stimulants such as coffee, alcohol and sugar. During such times, even if you cannot eat perfectly, it is imperative that you look at supplementation options to get you through the stressful period (see chapter 6).

Itchy skin and redness of the skin often relate to an overload on the liver. Chinese medicine recognises the relationship between red skin and too much heat in the body. Acidic foods need to be cut back, and omega 3 and 6 oils combined with a liver tablet are very useful in helping restore the skin to its normal state.

Creams such as sorbolene or a good basic moisturiser are helpful used on a daily basis, especially in colder climates or if you swim regularly in chlorinated pools. Creams made from chamomile are useful for shaving rashes. But unless you are attending to the internals of you skin condition no cream will work wonders.

As a general rule, always use a sunblock, and wear a hat when playing sport or at the beach as many men are prone to skin cancer. Make sure your doctor examines any unusual moles yearly. You can't be too careful.

✳General skin complaints

It is common to suffer dry skin through dehydration associated with travel. Some men are prone to dermatitis, where skin rashes may appear and are sometimes itchy.

On the extreme end of skin complaints is psoriasis. This is a dry, usually circular rash made up of patches of red skin covered by a flaky white build-up. It can be very itchy and often appears on elbows, hands and knees. Unfortunately for sufferers of this condition it doesn't look very attractive and can be very embarrassing in severe cases.

Treatment & prevention program

- For all skin conditions, use sorbolene cream daily (however, this does not allow you to forget the internal treatments).

- Swimming in salt water can clear dry skin rapidly and some exposure to the sun will give the skin the vitamins A and D it needs to heal and rejuvenate.

- Include a carrot juice daily for natural vitamin A.

- Eat tinned tuna, sardines and salmon at lunch rather than red meat in your sandwiches.

❊   Drink a glass of water every day for each glass of alcohol you take.

Supplements

❊   For mild cases of dry skin, take two omega 3 oil capsules daily. Include deep-sea fish in your diet three times a week and cut back on sugar, alcohol and junk foods. Make sure you rehydrate your skin by drinking eight to ten glasses of water daily. Keep a jug of water on your desk, or a teapot of tea such as my Triple E (liquorice-based), which is very helpful as a mild anti-inflammatory for the skin.

❊   For itchy dermatitis or eczema take high doses of omega oils – three capsules twice a day until improved. Include two anti-oxidant tablets (A, C and E vitamins); increase the dose to two tablets twice a day if the condition is bad.

❊   Take one vitamin B capsule a day as skin conditions often flare up under stress when adrenal glands are working overtime.

- Include a vitamin E tablet daily – 500 IU or double if you have very dry skin (use even if you are taking an anti-oxidant tablet).

Supplements for psoriasis

- Three capsules of omega 3 oils twice daily long term, even when the condition improves.
- In sufferers of this condition, the liver often needs assistance and the herb St Mary's thistle taken twice daily is effective.
- Liquorice tablets (two daily) and ointment (daily) are of great assistance to men who suffer psoriasis. If you are not taking capsules, then drink Triple E tea three times daily.
- If you suffer skin rashes when your immune system is lowered, include echinacea tablets: two a day for three months, then stop for six weeks. This is very useful in winter.

Groin rash

An itchy groin can be most annoying and embarrassing for men of all ages. It often comes about in hot weather.

Treatment & prevention program

- Always wear cotton underpants and take lukewarm showers. It can also be helpful to swim regularly in salt water.

- Include essential fatty acids in the form of omega 3 and 6 in your diet: take two capsules, twice a day.

- Creams generally do not work for this condition but if it is caused by a fungus, ask your doctor for an appropriate cream.

- Take two multivitamin tablets daily to ensure you receive adequate nutritional supplementation, especially if you suffer from poor digestion.

✳ Dandruff

Dandruff is an irritation and scaliness of the scalp. Dry skin flakes off and the scalp can become very itchy and inflamed. The condition can worsen with heat. It is usually caused by problems with the liver.

Treatment & prevention program

❊ Lower your intake of alcohol and saturated fats, and drink ten glasses of water daily.

❊ Try using a tar-based shampoo (available from your health food store) which can also be very helpful.

Supplements

❊ Include some essential fatty acids in the form of omega 3 and 6 capsules to give moisture to the skin. Take two capsules after each meal and reduce the dose when the condition improves.

- A liver detoxifying tablet is essential. St Mary's thistle is an excellent choice – take one tablet twice daily.

- An anti-oxidant with vitamins A, C and E, twice a day, is also useful.

✳ Balding

Balding is generally a hereditary condition but sometimes the loss of hair increases with stress. Men's responses to baldness vary enormously, in some cases affecting their body image and self-esteem. But there are ways of treating it.

Treatment & prevention program

I recommend taking a complex B vitamin tablet (two a day containing 50–100 mg of the main B vitamins, plus 50 mg of folate) and a *Ginkgo biloba* tablet twice a day. This herb increases circulation to the brain, and the better the blood flow and circulation, the better the growth of hair.

9
The brain

*Brain power

Diet and exercise fads come and go but one thing is for sure in relation to our ageing population: brain power is becoming increasingly important. Preventative health for this amazing organ will be a top priority for medical research over the coming years. Certainly, in the last sixteen years of my private practice I have seen both subtle and very substantial changes in men in relation to concentration levels and brain energy when their diet has been modified and certain 'brain foods' highlighted.

I have especially noticed much positive feedback from men when I have supplemented their busy lifestyles with some particular vitamins and herbs that have been used traditionally for increasing levels of oxygen to the brain. There is still so much information to be gathered and tested, but the following advice could be extremely helpful in improving the quality of your brain power.

Dr Darma Singh Khalsa, in his book *Brain Longevity*, talks about the good news of cognitive powers. He says that approximately half of all cognitive problems in men are not caused by Alzheimer's or age-associated memory loss, but by other factors, most of which can be avoided or compensated for. These factors include depression, strokes and general lifestyle factors.

Powerful stimulants such as alcohol, cocaine, marijuana and amphetamines all cause interference in the utilisation of acetylcholine, which is the most important neurotransmitter for memory. In fact, one of the characteristics of Alzheimer's is a marked deficiency in this important transmitter. It has now been found that even a moderate deficiency in some vitamins associated with acetylcholine can disrupt cognitive function. These vitamins include the Bs: B12, riboflavin and thiamine, which must be in adequate supply. B12 also helps to build the myelin sheath (the protector of the nerve cell) and prevents pernicious anaemia, which can rob the brain of oxygen. Folate is now also recognised as an essential part of the B vitamins for healthy neurotransmitters, especially in the prevention of Alzheimer's.

Minerals such as iron, iodine, zinc and copper are also

essential for good brain function. They can be found in high quantities in certain foods (legumes, green vegetables, sea vegetables, oysters, pumpkin seeds and wholegrain) and the addition of a good multivitamin tablet to your daily routine will ensure that they are always present in the system.

Oxygen is essential to the cognitive functions. Smoking, lack of exercise and poor diet contribute to a lack of oxygen in the body, which can become a problem for the brain.

Lead poisoning and exposure to mercury, along with exposure to pesticides and harmful sprays can also have a detrimental effect on the brain. If you have suffered from exposure to any of these elements, you should see a doctor or naturopath to find specific ways of assisting the body (especially the liver) to eliminate these heavy metals. A detox tablet for the liver made from St Mary's thistle and vitamins A, C and E is essential.

Food allergies can also disrupt your powers of concentration. The types of foods that may cause such a response include milk, wheat, refined sugars and packaged, commercialised foods which are often high in colourings and flavourings and low in nutrition. By following the diet for health and vitality as well as the treatment and prevention program, major allergies can be eliminated.

Treatment & prevention program

Following are critical dietary tips and supplements to obtain optimum brain power.

※ The brain must have sufficient supplies of oxygen to function effectively. Fatty foods deposit cholesterol and decrease the flow of blood carrying oxygen to the brain. What this means is that fatty foods must be cut back severely. They have been proven to cause hardening of the arteries and other cardio-vascular diseases as well. Fatty foods include:

- fried foods
- butter
- cream
- rich sauces
- hidden fat in refined and commercialised foods.

The motto is: *the fresher the better*.

※ Make sure you include fish that is high in omega 3 oils (this includes salmon, cod, sardines and mackerel) in your diet at least three times a week.

⚌ Avoid smoking and heavy drinking. These not only harden arteries but cause free radical damage to tissues in the liver as well as the brain. Remember brain cells cannot regenerate like liver cells. Just make up your mind to stop smoking. The chapter on giving up smoking in my book *Detox* may be helpful here.

⚌ Make sure you take regular holidays and find new ways to relax. High levels of continual stress produce stress hormones called glucocorticoids from the adrenal glands. These substances kill brain cells. Take up a new hobby or reorganise your work diary and block out a certain time daily just for you.

⚌ Don't get dehydrated. Not drinking water on a daily basis has been show to speed up the onset of Alzheimer's disease. Research carried out during post-mortems on Alzheimer's sufferers found that their brains were quite dehydrated. The brain 'dries up' without water. This means eight to ten glasses must be ingested daily; more if you play sport or work out. Many men in the 50-plus age group fail to make a concerted effort to drink water, fresh juice or herbal tea. Many of this

age group increase their alcohol, black tea and coffee intake –
all of which are dehydrating. They also fail to replace their
fluid loss with water after overindulgence in these
dehydrating beverages. Make sure you also include sea salt in
your diet to stop dehydration: half a teaspoon daily.

- Eat regularly. Not eating three proper meals a day can result
in very real problems with sugar imbalance generally, which
can affect the brain quite markedly. The brain needs good
quality, consistent levels of sugar to function – not hits of
sugar irregularly via coffee loaded with two to three
teaspoons of sugar; or alcohol; or a block of chocolate in place
of a regular meal. Good quality simple carbohydrates, from
fresh fruits and fresh juices, and complex carbohydrates, from
grains such as rice, couscous, grainy breads and steamed
mixed vegetables, are essential for brain power.

- Exercise regularly. Exercise improves oxygen levels in the
brain by increasing the supply of oxygenated blood, and
increases the levels of serotonin, the feel-good hormone that
prevents depression and keeps you inspired. An hour's

exercise daily is essential to good health. Some of that hour must be devoted to an aerobic form of activity that raises your pulse rate. This could be in the form of a four to five kilometre walk daily, swimming, bike riding, aerobic gym work or rowing.

- Make an effort to try new things. Brain cells need continual challenges and mind games. The brain needs exercise like all muscles and cells of our body. Try new brain challenges such as puzzles or word games, or study something completely new and different. For example, if you love languages then try studying something unrelated such as history or wildlife; or even something aesthetically interesting like colours or design; try mathematical studies if you don't have a head for figures. Take up flying or engineering or anything that changes your outlook and broadens your knowledge. Remember the process of using the brain is more important than the outcome – so you do not have to give yourself a hard time if you are not a famous pianist, painter or mathematician by 80!

Supplements

⚹ *Ginkgo biloba*: one or two tablets of the pure herb each morning. Repeat the dose later in the day if you are working long hours. Consult your naturopath, pharmacist or health store about a good quality tablet. It has assisted a number of my clients who work long hours and who need to apply strong powers of concentration daily. As ginkgo stimulates the brain, do not take it less than four hours before retiring, as it will tend to keep you awake, but when you have to work extremely long hours, a ginkgo tablet every three to four hours can be extremely helpful. Take it for at least three to four months to see how it can assist your concentration and sense of general wellbeing.

Ginkgo (*Ginkgo biloba*)

Ginkgo biloba is a herb that has been used worldwide for increasing circulation to the extremities of the body including the hands, feet and brain. Because of this action, it is also terrific for enhancing brain activity. The ginkgo is a deciduous tree that has been around for 150 million years. The green leaf that comes from this tree is a wonderful treatment for problems of memory, tinnitus, dizziness and the effects of high altitude. It can also help prevent stroke.

Ginkgo is especially useful for treating the early effects of dementia. I use it frequently to enhance memory, particularly in the 50-plus age group. If you are using aspirin or warfarin, check with your doctor before taking ginkgo.

Many other supplements have a general positive effect on good health but also specifically target the brain.

- Coenzyme Q10: 60–100 mg each morning; double the dose if you are going through a heavy work program for a few months. This anti-oxidant boosts oxygen levels to all parts of the body and repairs free radical damage. This supplement is particularly good for those who have suffered from chronic fatigue and have not fully regained their health.

▓ Two B complex tablets each day with 50–100 mcg B12 and folate. Recent research suggests that they are essential for healthy arteries. When the arterial blood is constricted, then fogginess, vagueness and sudden mood changes can happen, even if you have lots of sleep and a good diet.

▓ Vitamin E is found in avocado oil and other vegetable oils, especially wheat germ oil. This anti-oxidant vitamin assists in heightening energy due to its powerful effect on neutralising free radicals in the body. Using these oils on salads is a good idea; but it is generally not a high enough daily dose to assist the movement of oxygenated blood to brain cells, which ensures alertness of the brain. Take 500 IU daily to improve alertness.

▓ A Siberian ginseng tablet will help your system adapt to high levels of stress. Take one tablet twice a day during times of high stress.

▓ There are other anti-oxidants that you may wish to include in your daily regime. This really depends on how dedicated you are to achieving increased health and vitality with extra brain power. These include: green tea, grapeseed oil, turmeric, bacopa and schisandra. Sometimes you may find these extra herbs combined in a good quality anti-oxidant tablet: take one or two a day. One glass of red wine daily or two every second or third day is also acceptable.

- Omega 3 and 6 oil capsules, two to four capsules daily.

✳Ageing and dementia

Brain cells do not regenerate; therefore it is imperative that dementia is prevented as much as possible during the ageing process. Like most other diseases of ageing, dementia is also linked to the ingestion of toxic foods, cigarette smoking and overuse of alcohol. Excessive use of these substances causes long-term free radical damage to cell tissues, including the DNA of cells. The diet for health and vitality (see chapter 12) and daily ingestion of omega 3 and 6 oils are essential as preventative measures.

Supplements

The following supplements are vital for longevity and brain alertness after the age of 50 to 60.

* If a blood test shows elevated levels of the toxic amino acid (protein) called homocysteine, then vitamins B6, folic acid and B12 must be taken. These vitamins have the ability to lower homocysteine levels, especially in the elderly. A 5 mg folic acid tablet daily will lower homocysteine levels. As a general dosage, I recommend 400 mg of folate with 400 mg of B12 for men who eat poorly as well as for men over 50.

> **Brain food**
>
> Beef, liver, spirulina, kombu, milk, eggs, salmon, tuna, brewer's yeast, lima beans, soy beans, wheatbran, chickpeas, spinach, broccoli, avocado, bananas and turmeric.

* Blood flow to the brain can be enhanced through the two herbs ginkgo and bacopa. Buy a standardised extract of these herbs and take two a day.

- The aromatic root turmeric, so widely used as a food flavouring in India, has been found to be one of the most brilliant natural antidotes to free radical damage with regard specifically to dementia. In research in a village in India, none of the elderly occupants was found to have dementia and they all used this spice daily as a food source.

Meditation

Meditation is not a religion. It is a way of stilling our overactive brains and keeping them healthy. It has now become a great tool used by many top executives, politicians and other people who realise the great benefits of allowing the brain to slow down and stay in a state of relaxation for at least 20 minutes a day.

Many men use relaxing sports such as fishing, sailing and swimming as a form of meditation. Unfortunately, most of us can't do these sports often enough and therefore we need something else to fill the gap.

How does meditation work? The brain is powered by electricity. Every second trillions of brain cells fire electrical impulses that organise themselves into the following rhythmical patterns.

- Beta waves. The most common and highest frequency electrical impulses, which are firing during every waking moment. These waves are also associated with anxiety. In fact, when the brain spends a lot of time in the beta state we often refer to the feeling of being blocked, anxious and stuck in a problem.

- Alpha waves. These are slower and occur when we are relaxed: times such as during a pleasant walk or when you simply feel 'laid back'.

- Theta waves. These impulses are about two to four times slower that beta waves and occur during the meditative state, which is a state between wakefulness and sleep. People who can access these waves often have better problem-solving abilities and achieve deep and personal insights. The great news is that theta waves are not confined to the formal state of meditation but are increased by that process. It has been found that by practising meditation twice a day for 20 minutes you will be able to experience periods through the day where your brain will go into this state for problem-solving or to gain an insight to a situation that you have been grappling with.

�֎ Delta waves. These waves are associated with deep sleep and are the slowest of all the brain waves.

There are countless books on methods of meditating but mediation is not a mysterious process. There are several styles but they all end up at the same place. Choose whichever suits you: as long as it brings about a relaxation response in which your brain is floating in the theta state. The more you practise meditation, the more long-term benefits you will enjoy. It will positively affect every aspect of your health, brainpower and creative inspirations.

A method of meditating

Find yourself a quite spot and a comfortable position, possibly sitting cross-legged or on your knees. Try to still your mind and use your breathing to help yourself relax. In any form of meditation you will have many thoughts passing in and out of your brain. Try to ignore them. In the early stages use a word (or mantra) such as peace, relax, love, or one that may have significant spiritual implications for you. Keep rhythms of inhaling and exhaling steady – this is quite important.

Yoga is another way of meditating. This form of exercise combines the balancing of the body and the mind through breathing techniques, as well as strengthening the muscles and joints of the body. Sometimes you may wish to adopt a relaxation technique that yoga classes often use towards the end of the workout. You lie down and close your eyes. Focus on relaxing each part of your body from your feet to your head or vice versa. Relax each muscle group as your mind moves from each specific area. You can then repeat the relaxation again from the head to the feet.

A deeper form of relaxation

Sit in a comfortable position with your back straight and your legs crossed if possible. Put your hands in your lap with palms up; right hand resting on left with both thumbs touching.

Close your eyes and focus on letting go of all tension in the body through your breathing. Inhale deeply and hold the breath for 10 seconds and exhale. Repeat. Now just breathe in and out, in for about three seconds and out for the same time saying to yourself, relax. Focus your mental energy on the point between your eyebrows and top of your nose.

A mantra (or simple word, as already described) can be used or you can simply focus on your method of breathing. This breathing can only be done for about 10 minutes and then slow breathing can follow.

This deep relaxation method is effective in relaxing the brain and obtaining theta wavelengths. It's very useful for stress and can be used when you are working long hours and do not have the time to exercise to wind down and relax.

I suggest to many of my clients that they incorporate both forms of meditation into their life. You don't have to be a guru to practise basic meditation: 10 to 20 minutes once or twice a day will help you to manage stress very effectively. The rewards will astonish you.

10
Preventing cancer

There are many men who ask me what to take as a supplement to prevent cancer in general. This is a difficult question to answer, as we still do not fully understand the workings and intricacies of cancer in many cases. Certainly there are now established links between smoking, exposure to toxic substances and pesticide sprays, the high consumption of alcohol and cancer. There are also genetic links, especially in relation to prostate cancer and bowel cancer. Long-term stress, obesity, radiation exposure, hormonal imbalance and deficiencies in nutrients have all been linked to cancer too.

There are now active ingredients in certain herbs and foods that have anti-carcinogenic properties. I highly recommend you incorporate them into your diet on a regular basis. It is also wise to take one or more of the following supplements if you have had exposure to the any of the risk factors.

Treatment & prevention program

- Examine the diet for health and vitality in chapter 12. It is high in anti-oxidant foods, which have been shown to help prevent cancer. Incorporate this into your everyday life, along with some form of exercise and relaxation such as meditation for 20 minutes a day.

- An extract of green tea (*Camellia sinesis*) contains an active anti-tumour agent called epigallocatechin gallate. Take two tablets, two to three times a day, of the recommended dose of the standardised extract (5 g).

- A lycopene extract, which is made as a standardised extract from tomatoes, has been found to be a powerful anti-oxidant and has specific anti-cancer properties in relation to prostate cancer. A tablet should contain around 20 mg of lycopene: take one to two tablets a day.

> ### Lycopene
>
> Lycopene is a red carotenoid that gives tomatoes their
> colour. Unlike many other carotenes, lycopene cannot
> be converted into vitamin A. Instead it accumulates in
> various tissues of the body, especially in the prostate
> and the testes where it exerts its anti-oxidant effect.

- Other anti-oxidant/anti-cancer foods and herbs are rosemary, turmeric, flaxseed oil, selenium, fish oils, vitamin E, coenzyme Q10, and vitamin B12 with folic acid. You can obtain tablet forms of most of these substances; ask you naturopath for the dose suitable for your needs.

- An anti-oxidant herbal tablet made from St Mary's thistle, turmeric, rosemary, grape seed and green tea is a must for my cancer patients.

- After any cancer treatment, keep the immune system boosted by such herbs as astragalus and cat's claw.

Chemotherapy

If you are undergoing chemotherapy treatment, it is advisable not to take any anti-oxidants or anti-cancer supplements as they exert such a powerful influence that they can actually stop the chemicals from penetrating the cancer. You can take these substances after treatment or as a preventative before treatment. Always check with your doctor or health professional if you're unsure.

11
How to eat

✳Eating out

With hectic lifestyles, long working hours and social functions, eating out can become a treadmill of rich foods, indigestion and sleepless nights from over-consumption. In general, eating out can be a health hazard that becomes impossible to avoid.

Many men ask me how to choose from a menu when eating out to ensure good nutrition (and maintain vitality) without sacrificing taste. Following the simple principles below can help you to survive the restaurant scene and still enjoy the social benefits.

※ If you are not eating until late, try to eat a snack before you go out, preferably a protein snack such as some tuna on a slice of bread, soup, or even a milkshake with added protein in the form of whey powder. This will prevent you eating lots of bread when you arrive or eating fat-filled canapés. It will also help you to avoid drinking too much wine or beer before eating, which will heighten your cravings for food before the evening has even begun. This process is particularly important to follow before a cocktail party after work, for example.

* Pace your drinking by ordering gin and tonic or campari and soda or vodka and tonic before you go onto wine. There is less sugar in these drinks and your weight will be controlled more without the refined sugars of wine and beer.

* Always drink water with your wine and ask for some lemon to squeeze into the water. This helps digestion.

* Choose an entrée that has some form of protein, as you do not know how long the main dish may take to serve. There will be a temptation to eat lots of bread and drink more wine in between courses if you are very hungry. Minestrone soup, or a fish, chicken or duck entrée are ideal and will take longer to digest while you are waiting for your main course. Try and choose an entrée that is not filled with fat or fried.

- A raw salad with a protein is always useful at the beginning of a meal to get the digestive juices working well. This follows the same principle as a bitter drink: traditionally, a bitter drink such as campari and soda is taken before a meal to stimulate the digestive organs to better assimilate the meal to follow.

- If you are watching your weight do not eat bread. If you must, eat a bowl of steamed vegetables with your entrée instead of bread. Keep the olive oil dips and butter away from the table. They are too tempting, especially if there is a delicious crusty loaf sitting there as well!

- When choosing a main dish, lean towards a protein: fish, chicken, red meat (only twice a week) or legumes with added vegetables. Choose one carbohydrate like potatoes or rice and make sure you have both cooked and raw vegetables to both maintain health and satisfy hunger. I notice that if men just order a protein and salad without any carbohydrate or vegetables, they often then fill up on dessert as they are still hungry. The body is then overloaded with refined sugar that will not only cause weight gain but often disrupts sleeping.

- ▓ Always ask the waiter to make sure your food is not swimming in butter and oils. Your salads can be dressed with olive oil and lemon. Your vegetables can be steamed or oven-roasted.

- ▓ Do not eat fried foods such as chips, fried fish and duck in heavy oils. Do not eat the skin of chicken, duck or turkey as the skin contains the most fat.

- ▓ If eating out in a Thai or Japanese restaurant, make sure you do not eat lots of white rice (carbohydrate). Always choose protein and lots of vegetables on the side to satisfy the hunger and feed the system with anti-oxidants from the assortment of vegetables.

- ▓ When choosing a dessert, go for something that is not high in fat and sugar, preferably something with fresh fruit. Once a week, treat yourself to an decadent dessert if you must; but remember that if you do this too often you may notice a tendency for high triglyceride-induced tiredness the next day. All refined sugars, including wine, are classed as refined carbohydrates, which when overused will cause free radical damage leading to acute and chronic diseases. Alternatively, treat yourself to a small chocolate after dinner if you have chosen well with the rest of your meal. A small amount of sugar can be used as a treat, not as filler for a still-empty stomach.

※ Drink a pot of loose-leaf organic herbal tea after dinner, especially chamomile, peppermint or even my organic herbal teas such as Summer Delight, Petal or Apres. These are all wonderful aids for digestion before bed.

✳Takeaway food

※ Do not choose a heavy pizza before bed, especially if you are trying to lose weight. You are better off choosing Thai or other Asian dishes featuring fish, chicken, meat or tofu with vegetables and a little rice.

※ Equally, do not choose Indian food for a meal late in the evening. The sauces are very rich and your digestive system will still be going in the middle of the night while you are struggling to sleep.

▓ The best takeaway for health is a simple Thai meal, a light Chinese meal (no MSG) or a bowl of vegetable or minestrone soup.

▓ Try and include some of the anti-oxidants in your food, such as garlic, turmeric, rosemary, orange vegetables and of course some green vegetables.

▓ Ask for fresh herbs – mint, rosemary, parsley, thyme, coriander – in salads to help your digestion.

✳ Cooking at home

Many of my male patients confess that they have no idea how to throw a healthy meal together. For that reason, they tend to favour takeaway food as it is easy and requires no cooking apart from reheating in the microwave. Unfortunately takeaway food is often loaded with fat and, when reheated, many of the enzymes so essential for vitality are destroyed.

Over the years I have given the following hints to men, especially those who are bachelors or divorced, to help them prepare and cook a simple meal.

❖ Try and keep some healthy food in your cupboard so you don't get caught snacking on unhealthy options at midnight when you're hungry and tired.

❖ Go to the supermarket and buy the following pantry items that can be kept for long periods in your cupboard. These foods mean you won't need to shop every day, but only every two to four weeks:

- tins of salmon and tuna
- rice (preferably brown)
- cous cous
- pasta
- baked beans or a few tins of beans that you enjoy
- cereal
- tomato paste
- snap-frozen peas or some snap-frozen mixed vegetables of your choice
- sea salt, black pepper.

- Once a week, buy some fish, chicken or red meat and freeze. If you know you will be home for dinner, take the meat from the freezer in the morning. It's best that you buy or pack in small servings. Choose pieces of chicken or a small rack of lamb or a beef roll that is quick to cook in the oven. On the way home from work, buy fresh salad or fresh vegetables that you can steam. Avocados are always useful, as are eggs. Try to mix fresh foods with frozen foods if you are strapped for shopping time. Fresh is better as a general rule, but in reality I know this is not always possible. As long as you apply this simple principle, you can always find something nutritious to eat.

The following are some simple ways of preparing your meal.

- Roast. The oven is easy to use. Use your protein of choice (such as rack of lamb) and add some potatoes, pumpkin and onions to the pan and roast while you watch the news. You can use a tiny bit of butter or oil, or nothing at all. Fish can also be cooked this way.

- Grill. You may like to grill a fillet of fish or chicken that you collect on the way home, steam some baby potatoes and add some frozen peas right at the end of the steaming process.

The main principle with grilling and baking or roasting is to use your protein with some steamed or baked vegetables, or a salad on the side in hot weather. A little carbohydrate in the form of some rice, potato or a little bread is okay.

- Stir-fry. Chop your fresh vegetables and chicken pieces. Heat a little oil and butter and stir-fry in a wok, frypan or skillet. A stir-fry can also be placed on some rice or cous cous and you may wish to use herbs, garlic, shallots or curry for taste. Curries or other spicy foods can give you a restless night.

If you are exhausted and can't round up the energy for cooking, here are a few options:

- Bake a potato in the microwave oven or oven and eat this with a tin of tuna or salmon and an avocado or some green salad.

- Make a salmon or tuna sandwich and add as many greens as possible.

* A tin of baked beans is better than nothing. Eat with a salad if you can. This is not perfect nutrition, but it's better than eating nothing or lots of fatty food before bed.

* Make a nicoise salad with two boiled eggs, a tin of tuna and rocket or lettuce of your choice. Then throw in some raw sliced onions and boiled new potatoes for a little carbohydrate.

* If the worst comes to the worst then you can always make a protein shake from skim milk or water, protein powder and fruit. I find that sports people and those who arrive home late and feel acidic in the stomach often choose this option. The soy protein powder or whey protein is quite gentle on the digestive system.

Although this all sounds very simple I am always amazed how many men ask me how to throw together a protein and vegetable meal without much cooking.

I would advise keeping pasta and noodles to a minimum. So many men eat pasta with a tomato sauce, which only sustains energy for a short time. If you feel like this once a week, then have it, but eat a healthy salad with tuna or eggs on the side for more nutrition.

Some schools of thought advocate no protein foods in the evenings. It is true that red meat is very heavy, so I would suggest you try to have white meats, fish and vegetarian proteins such as legumes more often in the evenings as they are easier to digest.

If you have eaten protein for breakfast and lunch and are not exercising greatly, then a plate of steamed vegetables in the evening is better. The only problem with this sort of evening meal is that you may be hungry within a few hours. Then there is a temptation to eat a lot of chocolate or ice-cream to satisfy your hunger. This is okay occasionally, but if you eat like this regularly then you will overload your system with sugar before bed and have restless sleep and an acid stomach.

12

Diet for health and vitality

The following is a suggested healthy eating plan for men. It will give you some ideas for choosing appropriate foods throughout the day to maintain your energy levels and provide you with all the essential requirements. I have included mostly simple meals that are quick and easy to prepare or purchase.

Men generally crave more proteins and carbohydrates than women and often reject women's tendencies to introduce more vegetarian foods and salads into their diet. Men often feel the need to supplement this kind of diet with 'fillers' – the breads, pastas and potatoes they've been used to eating in the past. Men still crave these foods and seem to feel satisfied only if they have these carbohydrates in their diet.

Including some carbohydrates is fine but you need to be sure you're choosing quality carbohydrate, such as wholemeal or grainy breads, or couscous and brown rice. Potatoes left in their jackets are a favourite with many men but should be accompanied by other vegetables and a good quality protein. Rice noodle dishes with plenty of vegetables are also a good option.

Thick soups in winter filled with grains such as barley, buckwheat or rice with split peas and lots of vegetables are also great 'fillers'. Whatever you choose, avoid resorting to pizza and other fast foods, which contain little nourishment and lots of unwanted fat, let alone the hidden preservatives and food additives to make you irritable along the way!

To begin the day

Always drink a large glass of water on rising in the morning. This flushes the system and the bladder thereby helping the circulation and preventing build-ups that would cause unwanted gallstones, and helping the prostate gland.

Breakfast

A proper breakfast should always be eaten to start the day and give you the energy and calories that you need to concentrate. This is especially important if you are doing physical work or working long days.

※ Make yourself a fresh fruit juice using orange, pineapple or a fruit blend of your choice. Mango and pear or mango and peach are great combinations. In winter, apple or orange are good options.

※ Healthy cereal and low-fat milk with some protein powder sprinkled on top is a good start. Follow this with either an egg or two (have two eggs every second day if you do not have a cholesterol problem) on wholemeal toast (no bacon except perhaps on weekends if your weight is okay); or an omelette with tomato or vegetables (leave out cheese if you are watching your weight). Omelettes can be made with the whites only if you have high cholesterol.

※ A simple on-the-go breakfast option is baked beans on toast, or a tin of sardines or some mackerel on toast. These contain omega 3, which is excellent for keeping cholesterol under control.

✂ A smoothie is a great choice if you're short on time or you've missed out on breakfast for some reason. It can be made from skim milk and a fruit of your choice. Just throw them in the blender with a tablespoon of a tasty protein powder and a tablespoon of psyllium husks (a fibre which assists bowel movement and cholesterol reduction). These shakes can be made at the office if you have not had the time at home.

Between meals

Drink a jug of fresh water (filtered) between breakfast and lunch, and between lunch and dinner, or have a pot of herbal tea such as peppermint, Triple E or Summer Delight to drink, hot or cold, throughout the morning. This is a lovely alternative to coffee, and is great to offer your colleagues and clients when they visit the office.

Lunch

✂ Choose a healthy sandwich (have two or three if you're hungry) made from a good quality bread (preferably with whole grains, not white bread). Filling options include: chicken, tuna, salmon, egg or beef with three different raw vegetables or more. Go for a variety of colours, such as tomato (red), beetroot (deep red), carrot (orange), lettuce or rocket (green), cucumber or potato salad (white). This provides a variety of anti-oxidants in your diet.

* For a hot lunch, fish or chicken are excellent choices. You might also consider some form of legumes; for example, lentil soup or a legume curry. Try to include a variety of cooked or raw vegetables and choose a variety of proteins across your week. It's best to avoid eating red meat daily due to its high uric acid levels.

* Pasta with a good quality protein on top, such as fish or meat, accompanied by a salad is always a good option.

* Noodles are another healthy choice but make sure you fill up on vegetables with your noodles, otherwise you might be hungry not long after eating.

* Soup makes a great lunch in the winter months. It not only warms you up, it's also a good way of getting more vegetables into your diet.

I always encourage my clients to vary their diet as much as possible and to try different foods to those they normally eat (see also chapter 11 on eating out).

Whatever happens, it's vital to have a lunch break and eat a proper meal to keep your energy levels up for a busy afternoon. A fruit salad will metabolise in 30 minutes as it is predominantly made up of sugar, and you will be left hungry and craving more unhealthy sugars late in the afternoon. Fruit can be eaten after a proper lunch.

Snacks between meals

For people who suffer from hypoglycaemia (low blood sugar levels), those who tend to graze or those who are trying to lose weight, snacks between meals can be very appropriate. Some suggested options are as follows:

- A handful of almonds and a small amount of dried fruit.

- A piece of fruit and/or yoghurt.

- Half a sandwich such as curried egg or tuna with tomato and chilli.

✂ A protein shake with low-fat milk (these can be prepared at the office).

✂ Miso, chicken, vegetable or minestrone soup.

✂ A rice ball with vegetables, obtainable at health food stores.

✂ A muesli bar or protein bar.

Dinner

✂ Choose a protein from the following list: fish, eggs, chicken, beef, legumes, tofu. Grill, casserole or bake. Choose three coloured vegetables to accompany it, preferably 50 per cent cooked and 50 per cent as a raw salad.

✂ A rice dish with a protein and three coloured vegetables. Salad on the side.

✂ A pasta with a protein; for example, bolognaise or seafood sauce (use cream sauces very moderately). Thai or curry spices with meat or fish could be used as a sauce with egg noodles.

✂ A legume dish with a variety of beans such as chickpeas, soy beans and kidney beans, mixed with sautéed vegetables and a spice such as ginger, chilli, garlic or all three.

Try to avoid eating a heavy meal late in the evening. You should aim to eat your evening meal approximately four hours before you go to bed (see chapter 2 on weight).

If you are trying to lose weight, a thick soup and a small serve of a protein plus salad is appropriate.

A note on desserts

Use desserts as a special treat once or twice a week. Otherwise stick to fruit and yoghurt after meals.

A note on coffee

A coffee once a day after breakfast to get your day going is fine for most men but do not become reliant on it for your energy kick. If you are tired then look into the reasons why. Coffee is not the answer to long-term lethargy. If you are suffering high blood pressure, heartburn or anxiety, you should keep away from coffee altogether.

A note on alcohol

Try to drink quality wines that contain few preservatives and additives. Wines assist in the digestion of food. It is only the excessive use that will cause you liver and general constitutional problems.

A note on tea

Black tea such as English Breakfast, orange pekoe and Earl Grey all contain some caffeine (half as much as coffee). It has been found that they do contain some anti-oxidants. Green tea, which has not been fermented like black tea, contains double the amount of anti-oxidants and some caffeine.

Herbal tea doesn't contain any caffeine and has numerous active ingredients that assist digestion, the nerves, the lungs and the cleansing of the blood. Water can cause bloating so herbal tea is ideal to drink any time of the day as the pure herb softens the water and has healing properties for the body.

Herbal teas can play an important role in preventative health. As a herbalist and naturopath, I have created a range of organic loose-leaf herbal teas. These special teas have a variety of benefits including assisting digestion, helping to soothe the nervous system, and assisting in carrying nutrients around the body and removing wastes from the blood stream. Selecting the herbal tea that is suitable for your complaint is important and you may use the following guide to help you:

- **Apres** contains chamomile, fennel, aniseed and peppermint. This tea is highly suitable for those who suffer anxiety, stress, poor digestion, heartburn and mild insomnia. Chamomile has traditionally been used to soothe colic, upset stomachs in adults and frayed nerves. Fennel, aniseed and peppermint all aid poor digestion and help calm an aggravated stomach.

- **Berry** contains hawthorn berries, elderberries and juniper berries. Hawthorn berry has a history of assisting circulatory problems. In recent times this berry has also been found to have anti-oxidant properties. Elder and juniper berries assist the sweet taste of this natural herbal tea.

- **Lemon Tang** contains lemon grass and peppermint. This tea is ideal after fatty meals to help in the digestive process. It is cooling and soothing in hot weather and assists with kidney function.

❖ **Petal** contains organic red clover, lemon grass, lavender, rose petals, chamomile and buchu. This tea assists in cleansing the blood. Red clover has been used throughout history as a 'blood purifier' and we are now seeing it being used as a great balancer for the hormonal system. Lemon grass and buchu assist in stimulating the kidneys and therefore work as a mild diuretic, relieving fluid retention. Lavender, chamomile and rose are known to be 'calmative' plants, relaxing and healing for those who suffer stress, anxiety and the general overload of 21st-century living.

❖ **Summer Delight** contains organic spearmint, peppermint, lemon grass and aniseed. This minty tea is ideal for helping to detox the digestive system by stimulating digestive enzymes and relaxing and calming the body. Peppermint has a long history of aiding the digestion of fish and meat dishes. This tea is ideal after any meal.

- **Triple E** contains liquorice root, aniseed, fennel and peppermint. This tea has a profound effect on the bowel and stomach, helping with sluggishness and heartburn. The healing effects of pure liquorice root as a mild anti-inflammatory have been well documented. Hence liquorice is used in most cough medicines and laxative medication.

How to buy supplements

There are some very simple guidelines which can be applied to choosing quality supplements. It is important to be aware of these guidelines to ensure that you do actually experience what good quality medicinal herbs and therapeutic vitamins can do for your vitality and ongoing quality of life.

There are so many brands of vitamins and herbs in health food stores and pharmacies – all of different qualities and prices – and it is very difficult to know what exactly you should buy. In this book I have given general dosages for each condition, so you know what to look for. However, I always recommend, if you do want to get the most out of supplements and complementary therapies, a visit to a qualified, registered naturopath, herbalist, nutritionist or health consultant.

Tell them as much as you can about your medical history and

lifestyle in relation to your health. Make notes before your visit. If possible have a complete blood test before visiting your health consultant, or take along your latest test results. Also take along any medication you are on, as well as any vitamins or complementary medicines you may have been taking. It is vital that your practitioner knows what medication you are on from your doctor so they can discuss any contraindications in relation to your vitamins and herbs. They can sort out if they are suitable in dosage and quality and also check on expiry dates.

Your practitioner is trained to know the correct therapeutic doses for you, depending on your condition, body weight and height. They also know which products have quality standards and in-depth sourcing standards. If you are buying some supplements and are unsure about the information on the label, you should ring the information line (the number should be on the label) to ask about the company's sourcing and quality control standards. If this information is refused, then do not buy the product and again see your naturopath or trusted health food store to guide you to suitable brands.

The key words to look out for on labels of herbal medicine are 'standardised extract'. The 'standardised extract' tells you how much of the active ingredient (the medicinal part) is present in that particular supplement. For example, a label for echinacea supplements should say that you are taking 600 mg of echinacea root, containing alkylamides 2.65 mg (the active ingredient). Research was carried out on several echinacea products in the market to see is they contained the active ingredient of alkylamides (from the echinacea root). Three products did not use the echinacea root at all and three other products did not contain any active ingredient. So be sure to check the label.

If you are taking any form of complementary medicine for the first time, start off by taking one thing at a time and see if there is improvement over a period of three weeks. You may then wish to introduce another recommended supplement for the next three weeks. If you feel no better there can be a few obvious reasons.

- You are not taking the prescribed dose in accordance with your practitioner's instructions or the advice on the label.

- If you are following correct dosages then the medicine is either not suitable or you need to give the medication another month to feel the effect. In this case you can check with your health consultant.

- If you have self-prescribed, the quality or quantity of the medicine may be incorrect for your body size and weight. You would need to check this with your health consultant.

If you do not feel well with any supplement, stop taking it immediately and check with your consultant. Remember that any concentrated medicine, whether pharmaceutical or complementary, generally needs to be taken with food. Also do not take medicines before bed unless prescribed that way. Vary your medicines. Have some as tablets, powders and liquids.

Conclusion

It has been said that the 21st century is the 'new age of enlighten-ment' and perhaps this is true. I am certainly seeing this with the changes in recent years in men's attitudes to their health and their interest in their physical and emotional wellbeing. Good eating, sensible supplementation and enjoyable forms of relaxation are now recognised by many men as the stepping stones to taking control of their lives.

There are so many demands on men today – financial, physical and mental – that you need to be in peak condition to deal with them all satisfactorily. I hope this book has given you the knowledge you need to achieve this.

Remember, you don't have to do it all at once. It's about being 90 per cent good and 10 per cent naughty. Then, once your sense of wellbeing takes hold, you will be free to enjoy great quality of life.

Index

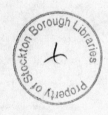